The Healthcare Appointment Playbook:

Understanding the System to Get the Care You Deserve

by

Barbara Alif Doran

Table of Contents

Your social history

Your family history

Your obstetric history

Your menstrual history

Sexual orientation and gender identity

Your sexual history

11. Your Vital Signs: Objective Information

Physical exam findings

Height and weight

Blood pressure

Pulse and respirations

Temperature

Last menstrual period

Pain levels

12. Objective Assessments: Tests and Screenings

Typical lab tests

Gynecology (well woman) exam test

Chronic illness screenings

Specific tests for individual health problems

Screening milestones

19. Rest

> Create a bedtime routine

> Slow down the pace of your life

20. Repeat

21. Resources

> List of questions to ask your provider

> Where to find health information

> Meal planning template

Citations

Acknowledgments

About the Author

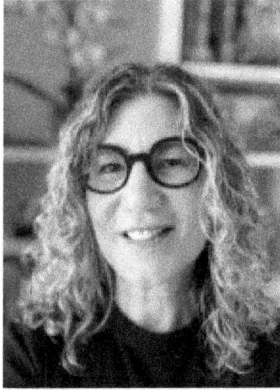

Barbara Alif Doran has always been driven by her passion for helping others. Initially considering a career as a math teacher, she later pursued a BA in psychology from Canisius University. Inspired by her late mother, a physician who appeared to her in a dream, Barbara changed course and earned a BSN in Nursing from the University at Buffalo. Despite initial hesitations, she pursued a master's in nursing degree specializing in Nurse Midwifery from the University of Pennsylvania.

Since 2001, she has been providing primary and well-woman care in Chicago at the same practice. Although she no longer delivers babies, she now cares for the women she helped bring into this world. Wanting to improve health equity and reduce health disparities, she earned an MBA from the University of Illinois at Urbana Champaign. She aims to have a greater impact on the health of others through her writing.

Barbara enjoys traveling, reading, and cooking. She lives in Chicago with her husband and their cats.

Introduction

health care or healthcare noun[1]

ˈhelth-ˌker[2]

: *efforts made to maintain, restore, or promote someone's physical, mental, or emotional well-being especially when performed by trained and licensed professionals.* – Merriam-Webster dictionary

I have probably never met you, but I care about you. Like the thousands of patients I have cared for over my career, I believe you deserve to live a healthy life and feel good while doing so.

I am an Advanced Practice Registered Nurse/Certified Nurse Midwife working on the Southwest Side of Chicago and I have been working in healthcare since 2001. I have taken care of generations of women from the same families and am now caring for patients who I helped bring into this world.

Through experience, I know that good care (and some luck) determines your health and wellbeing and your life expectancy—the age you are supposed to live to. Too often, I have witnessed patients receiving bad care, and I do not want you to become a statistic. I do not want you to develop a preventable condition like diabetes or heart failure because you were not taught how to prevent these diseases. I do not want you

---

1. **https://www.merriam-webster.com/dictionary/noun**

2. https://www.merriam-webster.com/dictionary/
health%20care?pronunciation&lang=en_us&dir=h&file=healthcare_1

to die a premature death because you don't know how to manage your health.

In this book, I am going to give you that knowledge. Please think of me as your health teacher. Your report card is your health record (which reflects your past and current health status). The grades you get going forward are up to both of us.

Knowledge fosters growth

When you understand what it means to be healthy and how to get there, you have the best chance of achieving and maintaining wellness, lowering your health risks, and living a long and full life in optimum health—physically, mentally, and emotionally. The mission of this book is to empower you to get what you need from every healthcare visit, especially your annual wellness checkups, and take control of your health with all the information, tools, and resources you need to thrive.

This book focuses on outpatient or ambulatory healthcare—the care you receive when you make an appointment at a clinic or medical office. In medical lingo this is called primary care. That's because, to prevent illness and hospitalizations, the most important healthcare work happens in primary healthcare provider offices. In the words of Benjamin Franklin, "An ounce of prevention is worth a pound of cure." I want to prevent you from needing acute or hospital care—unless it is necessary and for nonpreventable reasons.

I will also share behind-the-scenes information to help you better understand why we, your primary healthcare providers, do what we do (really, it's not a big secret). While this book doesn't directly address emergency room and urgent care visits, surgeries, or hospitalization, many of the things you learn here can be applied in those settings, too. Whether you're in a routine check-up or facing a medical emergency, you improve your outcomes when you know how to actively participate in your care.

Shared stories empower your health journey

Words will never express the gratitude I have for my patients, who have let me into their lives and shared their stories with me. This book is my gift to them and to everyone who doesn't feel seen or heard by their healthcare providers. I am going to share stories from my clinical experience (all names have been changed). You may recognize yourself in these stories because your life experiences may mimic those of countless people struggling with the same issues. You are not alone. Many others share your health challenges and feel similar frustration and vulnerability in a healthcare system that doesn't always support them.

If you are not ready to take control of your health, that's okay. This book will be here when you are. But here's the thing: based on my years of clinical experience, I know knowledge leads to positive changes in the way you manage your health. Many of my patients have thanked me for taking an uncommon amount of time to talk with them, teach them, and answer their questions. This should not be an exception, but the norm. Every visit you have with a healthcare provider should be constructive, where you are treated with dignity, and respect, feel heard, and have your concerns taken seriously.

So, if you are ready to learn how to be your own best healthcare advocate, keep reading.

Important Note

In this book, the word "provider" is used to speak about any healthcare provider you will interact with in primary care. This can be a physician/ doctor, advanced practice nurse/nurse practitioner, or physician assistant.

This book is geared towards women, because I am a women's healthcare provider. But many of the things I discuss relate to men as well. I use the words, "women" and "female," because the people I have cared for throughout my career have been women. But I understand that not all people assigned as female at birth identify as a woman and female. I do not mean to exclude people identifying as nonbinary, gender non-conforming, transman, transmasculine or transwoman.

Accessing Hyperlinks: This publication was initially released as an eBook and includes hyperlinks for accessing resources referenced throughout the text. For convenient access to these electronic resources visit https://www.barbaraalifdoran.com.

6

Chapter One

Healthcare Today: The Current State of Medicine

Today, we are living longer but are sicker and spending more money to remain alive. Healthcare is mentioned in the media daily. Experts and politicians discuss solutions constantly. But little is put into action and too often patients do not get the attention or care they deserve.

In a perfect world, the best health care is provided by a care team of healthcare professionals—a primary care provider and other related clinicians and technologists, which may include a dietician, mental healthcare provider, care coordinator, pharmacist, or community health worker. Together, these professionals combine their shared experiences and expertise to prevent chronic illness and diagnose and treat existing health issues.

The reality often falls short of this ideal due to provider shortages, professional rivalries, scope-of-practice disputes, and power grabbing. These conflicts can lead to fragmented care, communication breakdowns, and missed opportunities for collaboration, ultimately compromising patient outcomes and quality of care.

Our healthcare system—to put it bluntly—is screwed up. No one is denying this. Gone are the days when the majority of doctors knew their patients well and had long-term relationships with them. When medical decisions were primarily made by doctors based on patient needs, not insurance policies. When family medicine doctors were more common, handling a wide range of health issues before referring their patients to specialists.

These days, understanding health insurance feels like solving a complex puzzle. Navigating policies, choosing a suitable plan, and decoding co-pays, deductibles, and the maze of in-network versus out-of-network coverage can leave even the smartest people scratching their heads. Medical debt drives many into personal bankruptcy. The system uses confusing abbreviations and jargon that create unnecessary barriers. Terms like PCP, PPO, and HMO are a foreign language to most people, making healthcare feel like an exclusive club rather than a basic right. And that's before you get to prescriptions, inflated medication costs, and the long wait to see a healthcare provider—if you can find one taking new patients.

Since the Affordable Care Act (also known as Obamacare), health insurance has become more affordable. Although, I would argue that many of the most affordable plans on the insurance exchange have limited options for finding care. In my Southwest Side practice, I see patients who live in downtown Chicago because the providers closer to their homes can't afford to or refuse to accept their lower cost insurance plans. That's simply not right.

Provider shortages put a strain on care

There is a critical shortage of healthcare providers, especially in primary care where less money is made. (The money in healthcare is in specialty care.) Providers are going on strike or leaving the profession altogether, frustrated by working conditions. Some providers feel like they are suffocating at work and are doing their best to stay above water to keep breathing. Provider burnout is real. (I went through it myself, which is the reason why I wrote this book.)

This shortage is leaving a growing number of patients underserved—especially our aging populations—the sick ones and the ones not yet sick but requiring more preventive care. As healthcare providers come and go, you may not see the same person more than once or twice. From your perspective, this creates frustration and mistrust in the healthcare system. It is difficult to trust someone who you may never see again. You no longer have the opportunity to make long-lasting relationships, or if you have had that luxury, the provider you've seen for years may have just left the practice. As a result, you often have an incomplete health record.

Additionally, with too few primary care providers, you may not see a healthcare provider that looks like you and you may be hesitant to share your issues because you think they will not get you. And they may not— although, please note that a good healthcare provider will ask questions so they can get to know you and your concerns better.

Healthcare as a global problem

America is not unique. Healthcare systems around the world have significant challenges. Provider shortages are an issue in many countries. High blood pressure is common worldwide, called the silent killer, silently damaging heart, kidneys, and brain, leading to serious health problems like heart attacks and strokes. It is especially common in my patient population. Additionally, we have a maternal health crisis gripping many parts of the world, with the United States standing out as a particularly troubling example among developed nations.

While some countries have found effective ways to address these health challenges, others are falling way behind, creating a gap in the quality and accessibility of care.

Life expectancy is moving in the wrong direction

I hate to be Bad News Barbara, but health trends in the U.S. and worldwide are heading in the wrong direction. The average person in the US is supposed to live, on average, to 77 years of age. With good healthcare, they may live a decade or two longer. But because of a breakdown in our healthcare system over the past few decades, too many people are dying prematurely.

The differences in the US alone are especially concerning when broken down by race and ethnicity, as the chart below—Life expectancy at birth, by Hispanic origin and race: United States, 2019-2021—demonstrates. The gap in healthcare quality and access is widening, creating a stark divide between those who receive top-notch care and those left struggling in underserved areas, often separated by just a few zip codes or income brackets.

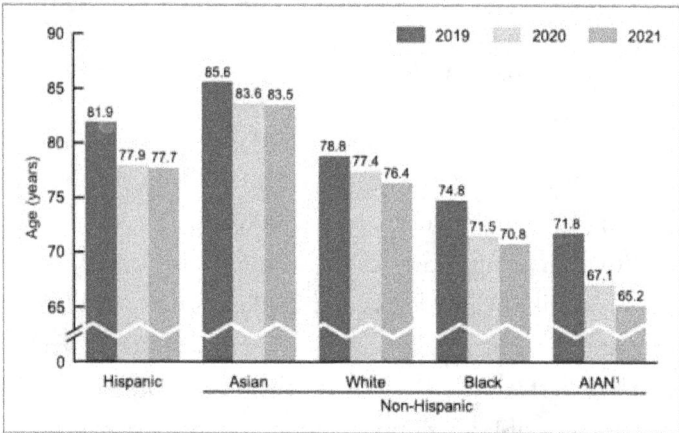

[1] American Indian or Alaska Native.
NOTES: Estimates are based on provisional data for 2021. Provisional data are subject to change as additional data are received. Estimates for 2019 and 2020 are based on final data. Life tables by race and Hispanic origin are based on death rates that have been adjusted for race and Hispanic-origin misclassification on death certificates; see Technical Notes in this report.
SOURCE: National Center for Health Statistics, National Vital Statistics System, Mortality.

Consider people in your life who you were told died of "natural causes." If they were below their 77-year life expectancy, their death was not natural but premature. Some illnesses are genetically related. Some may result from environmental factors. But the majority of chronic illnesses that cause premature death can be prevented or managed with proactive healthcare.

The business of health: profits versus prevention

The primary care you receive should emphasize preventive care. However, many providers have not been trained in prevention and provide sick care rather than health and wellness care. There is a power play going on between large healthcare systems and insurance companies who pay for health services. Today, both operate with a profit motive, often at odds with their advertised humanitarian visions. Insurance companies make money when they collect more in premiums than they spend on care. A quick internet search reveals the billions of dollars large health insurers make in profits, creating stress for all stakeholders in healthcare (hospitals, providers, patients, and pharmacies). While insurers encourage yearly preventive health checkups, this is largely to avoid paying for more expensive treatments later, not because they care about the people they cover.

The rest of the healthcare system—hospital systems, laboratories, and even some clinicians—too often views healthcare as a business rather than a public service or a fundamental human right. Prevention isn't as profitable as treatment because it reduces the need for costly interventions. Large corporate healthcare systems often make more money when people get sick, as illness creates the need for more visits, medications, treatments, hospitalizations, and surgeries. This profit-driven model can sometimes lead to overtreatment or unnecessary procedures, further driving up costs without necessarily improving patient outcomes.

Here is an interesting chart highlighting the costs spent providing care in the U.S. compared to similar countries without improving life expectancy.

Life expectancy and per capita healthcare spending (PPP adjusted), 2022

Country	Life expectancy	Health spending, per capita
United States	77.5	$12,555
Germany	80.7	$8,011
United Kingdom	80.9	$5,493
Austria	81.1	$7,275
Canada	81.3	$6,319
Netherlands	81.7	$6,729
Belgium	81.8	$6,600
Comparable Country Average	82.2	$6,651
France	82.3	$6,630
Sweden	83.1	$6,438
Australia	83.3	$6,372
Switzerland	83.6	$8,049
Japan	84.1	$5,251

Notes: Comparable countries include: Australia, Austria, Belgium, Canada, France, Germany, Japan, the Netherlands, Sweden, Switzerland, and the U.K. See Methodology section of "How does U.S. life expectancy compare to other countries?"

Source: KFF analysis of CDC, OECD, Australian Bureau of Statistics, Japanese Ministry of Health, Labour, and Welfare, Statistics Canada, and U.S. Office of National Statistics data • Get the data • PNG

We need to shift the focus back from profits to people. I want to see prevention become the norm. But for that to happen, it must begin with YOU, the patient. **If you are willing to take personal responsibility and learn the tools you need to advocate for your health and wellness, you can make a real difference.** This means asking questions about preventive measures, understanding your treatment options, and prioritizing lifestyle changes that promote long-term health. By becoming an informed and engaged patient, you'll be better equipped to navigate the complexities of healthcare, make smarter decisions about your well-being, and help drive a much-needed change in our healthcare system's priorities.

This book empowers you with the knowledge and skills to do that, helping you take control of your own health journey in a system that often feels overwhelming. In the process, you may also improve the health of your family and loved ones, becoming a role model for children, siblings, friends, parents, and coworkers.

Chapter Two

You Can Be Your Own Best Health Advocate

Too much of primary healthcare today is provider-driven, not driven by you, the patient, who is the customer. What do I mean by this? The expectation is that when you visit your healthcare provider for an issue, they will ask you questions, will let you ask questions, and will provide a solution for your health problem. More often, you'll find that they spend most of their time looking at a computer screen, rush you through the visit, and leave you with unanswered questions. You may worry your provider has experienced whiplash from entering and leaving the exam room so quickly.

If you're lucky, you may have a rock star for a healthcare provider (I know I do), a person who listens, does not judge, treats you with respect, takes your opinions into consideration when making a care plan, and reviews and updates your health history. (If you have that type of healthcare provider, let them know you appreciate them, because it will make their day, trust me.) Unfortunately, many providers are burdened by corporate health practices that give them little time to engage with patients fully. The average length of a patient visit in the U.S. is 15 minutes.

Some providers think they have all the answers, know what is best for you, and do not work with you to create your care plan. They want their visits with you to be quick and painless, like removing a band aid. I'm here to tell you that healthcare providers do not have all the answers. Just because we went to medical school, or graduate school to become a nurse practitioner/midwife or physician assistant, does not mean we know what is best for you. We are not living your life and without having a conversation and checking in with you, we do not know your fears and concerns. Because we make a recommendation, does not mean you have to do it.

To get the most from your provider visits and leave feeling confident you understand your options for managing your health, consider the following five tips.

1. Know your rights as a patient

Though I have spent my career working in communities of color, I'm white. Most of my friends are white and all of us have experienced struggles with the healthcare system. Too often my friends and their families feel like they are a nuisance to their providers rather than being valued. These frustrations with the system are widespread, but they disproportionately impact people of color and those living in rural areas, who often face greater challenges in accessing quality care.

Sadly, bias exists in the healthcare industry. Healthcare providers should never make assumptions about patients. Instead, as Ted Lasso would say, we should "Be curious, not judgmental" in our approach to patient care. This philosophy should guide every aspect of the visit, from our first impressions upon entering the exam room, through how we conduct the visit, ask questions, listen attentively, give patients opportunities to speak and ask questions, and create a plan that works for them.

Most healthcare providers attend a mandatory bias training every year and yet, you may have felt dismissed or disrespected because of your skin color, sexual orientation and identity, job title, where you live, or how much you make. You might feel that if you looked, acted, or lived somewhere different, you would be treated differently.

The truth is, when you learn how to take control of your healthcare experiences, you are in the best position to assert yourself and ask for better care.

As a patient, you have several fundamental rights that healthcare providers and institutions must respect.

- The right to be treated with dignity and respect
- The right to receive care without discrimination
- The right to privacy and confidentiality of your medical information
- The right to informed consent before any procedure or treatment
- The right to refuse treatment
- The right to access your medical records
- The right to receive clear explanations about your diagnosis and treatment options
- The right to participate in decisions about your care
- The right to seek a second opinion
- The right to file complaints about your care without fear of retaliation
- The right to be informed about the costs of your care

It's important to remember that you, the patient, make appointments to see us, not the other way around. While some providers attribute biased behavior to implicit bias (suggesting they're unaware of it), I challenge this assumption. People often sense when they're being judged. Many healthcare issues could be resolved if providers engaged in genuine conversations with patients rather than talking at you. **The solution is simple: providers need to treat patients the way we would want to be treated by our own healthcare professionals. In essence, we should practice the golden rule in healthcare.**

So, stand up for your rights when necessary. You should never feel they are being dismissed.

2. Don't let the provider rush your appointment

A 2017 report showed that primary care providers, on average, spend from 9 to 24 minutes with patients, affected in part by the reason for the visit and provider's specialty.[1] (Internists tended to spend more time than family physicians.) While some practices schedule 20 minutes for an established patient (established to the medical practice or to the provider) and 40 minutes (or more) for a new patient or annual wellness visit, too many limit visit time, to the detriment of the patient. In fact, a 2023 cross-sectional study of 4,360,445 patients found that shorter visits were more likely to result in inappropriate prescribing of medications.[2]

You may be thinking to yourself, "I have never had someone spend 20 minutes with me." Well, my friend, part of being treated with respect and dignity is being given the time you need to explain any health concerns you have and understand your treatment options. If you need more time, ask for it.

3. Insist on options

Healthcare providers are not your parents and should never take a "do it because I told you so" approach to healthcare. Healthcare providers often have a one size fits all approach to how they care for patients. A medication toolbox, so for diabetes, the provider always prescribes medication A, for hypertension/high blood pressure, medication B, maybe medication C. If a patient wants to start birth control pills, they prescribe medication D. These providers believe that rather than talking with patients about what happens in their lives, prescribing more medication will help (it often does not). They forget (or simply don't have time to care) that each person has different side effects. Too often they rely on medical research that has studied medication in just one population and prescribes it for another. Because one medication may work for someone without side effects does not mean it will work the same way for another. We are all unique.

There's never a one-size fits all answer to a health problem, and often there are many options for treatment. Your body. Your choice. Your health.

You shouldn't be intimidated by providers advanced degrees and job titles and afraid to ask questions. Not to burst the bubble, but we are human just like you. We have no superhero powers. The only difference is that we know more about health, medicine, and how the healthcare system functions than most of our patients. Truth be told, any healthcare provider, or human being for that matter, should be learning continuously. What we learned during schooling and training may have (most likely has) changed. The human anatomy remains the same, but managing chronic conditions has new options. New information is gathered at the speed of light. New illnesses like COVID emerge and old ones like polio and measles resurface. Because someone learned one way, they may continue to practice that way even if it is no longer correct. All healthcare providers have access to current evidence-based medicine, and all must do continuous medical education to renew their licenses to stay current with treatments and medications.

If you do not understand something or question what treatment options you're being given, speak up and ask. You may think you are annoying your provider, and truth be told, you may be. But tough. **Your visit is about you, not your provider!** In primary care, once you have been given your options, you should be given time to think about them and how they can affect you.

4. Request clarification

Providers often use big words and may explain things in ways you do not understand—this comes second nature to us and we often forget that our patients do not have the vocabulary and knowledge about healthcare related issues. It is our job to explain everything in understandable terms, not your job to figure out what we're talking about. We are your health educators, your teachers about all things related to your health and wellness, and it is our responsibility to explain things in ways our patients understand so you get good health grades.

I'm going to keep repeating this, because I think it's important. Your medical record is your report card. The grades you get (your health status) are dependent on both good teaching and also the effort you put into staying healthy. If you become sick with a preventable illness because your healthcare provider didn't properly teach you, then the system failed you. **If you fail because you were taught but did not make good decisions, following the care plan you and your provider made together (taking your life and its messiness into consideration), then you have failed yourself.**

When you are sick, managing your health status takes more than a simple prescription. You need to understand why you developed a disease or illness and how to improve the disease—or not make it worse—with lifestyle modifications and, if needed, medication. Medication is never the only solution to manage a health problem. The world you live in and what you do to your body (how much you move, what you eat, how much you sleep, rest and manage stress) affects everything about you, including your health.

5. Be as bold with your health as you are with your hair

To help illustrate how you can be an advocate for your own health, I'm going to compare your healthcare visits with a trip to a hair salon. Why? Because when you make an appointment at a hair salon, you're in control of the experience. When you go to the salon, the stylist doesn't prevent you from describing what style you want them to create for you. You sit in the chair, talk about your goals, and have a conversation about what will work best for your hair. You are paying for the stylist's service and expertise. Otherwise, you would do your own hair. At the end of your appointment, your stylist hands you a mirror to make sure you are satisfied and makes any adjustments necessary. You then pay for the service and leave, hopefully walking away feeling good about yourself and your hair.

The same should hold true in healthcare. Your interaction with your healthcare provider should be a dialogue—a conversation. You should be given the time to talk about your concerns, needs, and health goals. Your provider, who has specific expertise in healthcare, should give their opinions and offer suggestions based on your conversation, what they know about you, and their exam. They should also seek your input and get your commitment before implementing any treatment plan. Healthcare providers are trained in shared decision-making, but too many aren't given the time for collaboration. Therefore, you may need to stand up for your rights and demand it. **You should never leave a healthcare visit with unanswered questions and confusion about your own health.**

Oddly, if you're like many people, you may care more about your hair, nails, and outward appearances than your own health. When you feel well, your health is out of sight and out of mind. While you cannot see inward, if you listen carefully, you can feel both the signs of health and wellness as well as the symptoms of sickness. When you are in a good state of health and well-being, you feel good physically and emotionally. You have less aches and pains, and you are happier. You may only need an annual checkup to make sure there are no hidden health issues you need to address. But when you're feeling lousy and need the support of a healthcare provider, you (or your insurance company) pay for their services, just like you do for your hair stylist.

So, remember this: **You own your visit.** As the customer, you should be the most important person during the visit and the center of your provider's attention. Ask questions, be an active participant even if it feels awkward. If you feel rushed, slow the visit down by asking questions. **Come prepared to your visits with a list of your health concerns, either written on paper or in the Notes app in your phone.** That way, you'll have something to refer to in case you get confused, feel nervous, rushed, or intimidated.

If patients like you begin to speak up for what you want in terms of your healthcare and fill out patient satisfaction surveys after your visit (i.e. add a note about wanting more time and less rushed visits), I believe the system will change. There will come a day when providers are given more support so they can spend more time with their patients. This change is not going to come from healthcare administrators who are thinking about how much money they can make by filling providers' schedules with more patients. It must come from YOU, the patient.

Patients have a voice and it can be loud and impactful. It is too bad patients can't unionize to get the most from their healthcare experiences. That would really make a difference.

Patient Story

I have a patient, Anne, who I see every three months for her birth control injection. She is 31 and a former heavy smoker who still smokes but is cutting back. She has high blood pressure—consistently 150s/90s (normal is less than 120/80). She has a high body mass index (BMI) because she eats mostly fast foods and few vegetables and fruits, prepares few meals at home, drinks mostly water, sometimes juice, and does not drink alcohol or use any substances. She works at improving movement and rest, walking when she's at work and sleeping 7 to 8 hours each night. She has a strong family history of high blood pressure.

Anne has refused medications on many visits. I counseled her on her health risks and my concerns for her, given her persistently high blood pressure, lifestyle, and family history. We discussed things she can change (diet, smoking, activity) and things she can't (family history). I referred her to another provider at the clinic so she could get a second opinion. The provider prescribed medication, which Anne took multiple times but stopped because she did not like the side effects. She mentioned at a follow-up visit with the other provider, who simply refilled the same medication and called patient non-compliant.

When Anne came back to me for a scheduled visit, we discussed her concerns and I offered to start her on a different medication. She declined. Then, on another follow-up visit with me, her blood pressure was still elevated, despite trying to reduce salt from her diet and eat more vegetables, be more active on her days off by relying less on public transportation and walking more and limiting her smoking to 1 to 2 cigarettes per day. We discussed the fact she was doing all the right things, but with her family history, her blood pressure was still high. She agreed to start the different blood pressure medication after I explained the possible side effects. At her three-month follow-up with me, she'd been taking her medication almost every day and said she wasn't having any side effects. She continues with the same lifestyle changes and her blood pressure is controlled with the medication.

It took months of conversation for her to agree to take medication after expressing my concerns for her health. But it was her choice. Until she agreed to take medication, all I could do was write in my progress note about our discussion. This is shared decision-making. I may not like every care plan we decide on, but in this case, Anne trusted me enough to finally agree to take medication.

Take Note

Healthcare providers do more than see patients. Providers are often their own administrative assistants, putting in many hours of extra time they aren't paid for. They must answer and make telephone calls, fight with insurance companies to get referrals approved for their patients, answer patient messages in patient portals, review test results, talk to pharmacies about medication substitutions when an insurance plan suddenly stops covering a medication a patient has taken for years, and attend trainings/ meetings. While it shouldn't affect the time you have with your provider, too often it does. Knowing this may help to understand why your provider cuts your visit short or why you may not be able to see the same provider every visit.

Chapter Three

———

The Different Types of Healthcare Providers

What is a healthcare provider and why do I not use the term doctor?

Not every person who provides primary medical care is a physician/doctor. In fact, most states in the U.S. grant licenses to non-physician healthcare providers to practice independent of a supervising physician. These providers, also known as advanced practitioners, can collect health histories, perform exams, order labs and radiology studies (like blood tests, ultrasounds, x-rays, MRI), refer to specialists, and write medications just like doctors.

At a time when our healthcare system is coping with a shortage of physicians, non-physician healthcare providers increase access to primary care, especially in underserved areas. They often provide similar quality care at lower costs compared to MDs/DOs.

While many physicians have mixed feelings about whether advanced practitioners are qualified to provide care independently, believing that the best care is given under the supervision of a physician, generally doctors report having good working relationships with Advanced Practice Providers.

From my experience, just because someone went to medical school does not mean they are superior to healthcare providers who got their master's degrees or doctorates. For routine primary care, the exact credentials of the person you see is not as important as the quality, respect and care you receive from them. What's most important is that the healthcare provider is providing care within their scope of practice, treating you with dignity, respect and compassion—treating you the way they want to be treated by their own healthcare provider or the way they want their loved ones to be treated.

Specialty care and surgery is a different matter, but many specialty practices also employ non-physician providers to support physicians and interact with patients.

In selecting a primary care provider (PCP) to oversee your care, it helps to understand the backgrounds of each type of provider.

Types of providers

Physicians/Doctors

MDs (Doctor of Medicine) and DOs (Doctor of Osteopathic Medicine) are both licensed physicians in the United States who can practice medicine. They earn a bachelor's degree plus attend four years of medical school followed by three to seven years of training in a residency program, focusing on a specialty—from family medicine to dermatology to brain surgery. Both MDs and DOs can pursue the same specialties. Some physicians go on to more specific trainings for fellowships, but you may not interact with them in primary care. The difference between MDs and DOs is their philosophical approach to medicine. MDs practice allopathic medicine, which focuses on diagnosing and treating specific conditions. DOs practice osteopathic medicine, which emphasizes the body's ability to heal itself and takes a more holistic approach to patient care. DOs receive extra training in Osteopathic Manipulative Treatment (OMT), a hands-on technique to diagnose, treat, and prevent illness or injury.

Residents

These physicians have graduated medical school but are being trained in a particular area of medicine and often provide care alongside their attending physicians in large practices and teaching hospitals or academic medical centers affiliated with a university. In primary care, residents receive training in internal medicine, family medicine, pediatrics, and obstetrics/gynecology. Medical residents make up an important part of the healthcare provider labor force. (Until they complete their training, they do not earn the same salaries as attending physicians, so health systems benefit financially from having them on staff.) When a resident cares for you, they should introduce themselves as a resident physician. **Because residents are still in training, if you have any doubts about their diagnosis or treatment recommendations, you have the right to ask to speak with their attending physician.** Often, they will bring in the attending without having to be asked. This ensures you receive the best care from an experienced physician.

Advanced Practice Clinicians or Providers

Non-physician clinicians include Advanced Practice Registered Nurses (APRNs) and Physicians Assistants (PAs).

APRNs can practice as Nurse Practitioners, Certified Nurse Midwives, and Nurse Anesthetists (the latter work in inpatient/hospital systems and surgical centers, not in primary care). They first earn their bachelor's degree and registered nursing license (RN). Many work as RNs before going on to get their master's degree in a medical specialty. With this background in caregiving, many APRNs are more likely to emphasize whole person care and communicate health information in words you can understand easily. Some APRNs have a Doctor of Nursing Practice (DNP), which requires a year or two more education than a master's degree. APRNs in primary care specialize in adult and geriatric medicine, family medicine, women's health, pediatrics, and psychiatry. Advanced practice RNs are independently licensed providers. Some states require APRNs to work in collaboration or under the supervision of a physician. Currently, 28 states and the

District of Columbia allow APRNs to practice independent of a physician's supervision. In these states, APRNs can evaluate, assess, and diagnose conditions, prescribe medications, make referrals and bill for their services under their own license. They perform many of the same tasks that physicians do.

Physician Assistants must have a 4-year bachelor's degree before starting graduate school in general medicine. Their training is patterned after medical school education. A PA master's degree, which takes an average of three years to complete, can be either a Master of Physician Assistant Studies (MPAS) or Master of Clinical Health Services (MCHS). PAs must be supervised by physicians to some degree in every state in the US; but the amount of supervision varies from state to state. They can take health histories, perform physical exams, order screenings and lab tests, perform routine diagnostic tests, make diagnoses and referrals, and assist in surgeries. They can order medications authorized by a physician. In some states, PAs can open their own practice but still need to collaborate with a supervising physician.

You may also see students studying to be nurse practitioners and physician assistants. Students should introduce themselves as such. During your visit, you should also see their clinical preceptor (a practicing APRN or PA), who will make sure you have received the best care and all issues were addressed during your visit.

Chapter Four

————

Your Primary Care Provider (PCP)

Most healthcare plans either recommend or require you to have a PCP. Any of the healthcare providers noted in Chapter Three can serve as one. Your PCP serves as the director of your healthcare journey.

Most primary care MDs and DOs have certifications in family medicine, internal medicine, or pediatrics. Though most obstetrics/gynecology (OB/GYN) physicians consider themselves specialists, OB/GYNs are also capable of being your PCP. Family medicine doctors care for patients from birth through old age. Internal medicine doctors, also called internists, specialize in care for adults over 18. Pediatricians generally care for patients from birth through age 21, although some refer patients to a new provider when they turn 18. OB/GYNs care for all women's health issues. Some consider themselves specialists and only provide specific women's health care like well woman exams, reproductive, prenatal, and postnatal care. APRNs or PAs can also specialize in adult or family medicine, pediatrics, and women's health.

A PCP knows more about health, wellness, and the healthcare system than you, so it is their responsibility to teach and guide you. As I mentioned earlier, your medical record is your health report card. The grades you get regarding your health and wellness are up to you. But if you don't have good teachers, you may not earn good grades and your health may suffer as a result.

In previous decades, you might expect your PCP to manage your health for many years, maybe even over your entire adulthood. But with high provider turnover and burnout, this rarely occurs today. A provider may stay with a practice for several years, get frustrated, and move onto another practice. With high demand for PCPs in almost every region in the U.S., it's easy for them to relocate and leave you seeking a new provider.

It's hard to trust your provider when you see a different person each time or lose a provider you've known for years. This is a big problem in healthcare today. Profit-seeking healthcare organizations don't value patients enough to invest in keeping good primary care providers around. As a patient, you need to learn to demand more, which is why I'm giving you the tools to take charge of your health and get the best out of each healthcare visit, regardless of how long you have known your provider.

Finding the best PCP for you

You may go years without needing more than an annual checkup, but when you have a medical issue, you want a PCP in your corner you can trust to respect and meet your health goals.

A good PCP offers continuity of care, comprehensive health management, and personalized guidance that can lead to improved health outcomes, early detection of potential issues, and more efficient navigation of the complex healthcare system. In most Healthcare Maintenance Organizations (HMOs), you must see your PCP before you can get referrals for any specialty medical service.

Depending on your health insurance (see Chapter Eight for more information on types of insurance), you may be asked to pick a PCP within your insurance's network. Or your insurance company may assign a PCP for you. If you can afford it, you might consider a PCP in a concierge medicine practice, where you pay a membership fee for care throughout the year.

If you don't get to choose, you can use the tools you learn in this book to ensure you get the best care possible. Know that it's your right to change providers at any time. The challenge will be finding one taking on new patients.

If you get to choose your provider, ask family and friends for referrals and check online reviews. You can also check background credentials on the provider's practice website. Use your first "get to know you" appointment to ask questions about the provider's approach to care and evaluate how well they listen to your questions and answer them. Find out what healthcare network they are part of and if they have good relationships with other providers in the community. If they are a sole practitioner, who offers backup care? Do you feel confident they will honor your health goals and let you participate in your own care? Do they make you feel?

comfortable asking even the most intimate questions about your body and health?

You may not be able to choose your provider; but you can still get to know them at the first visit and ask the same questions. Personally, I have had patients who have seen other providers before seeing me, outright telling me about their bad experiences with other providers and that I better be different. To break the ice, I usually respond, "No pressure," but encourage them to tell me their concerns first before opening their electronic medical record.

If the first provider you meet with does not meet your standards for care and you have multiple options to choose from, don't hesitate to find another who does.

Chapter Five

―――

Proactive Health: The Power of Preventive Care

Healthcare is not limited to sick care. While it does include sick visits, which are critical for restoring good health, it also includes annual wellness visits to proactively manage your health and prevent future problems.

We all need to prioritize preventive care and regular check-ups to avoid the cascading negative effects of illness and ensure better overall health and life satisfaction. If you are healthy and do not have a chronic condition, this once-a-year checkup is your opportunity to understand your risk factors, receive education about preventing disease and illness, and get the screenings you need to maintain a state of wellness and live your healthiest life. If you are only engaging with the healthcare system for sick visits, you are missing a valuable opportunity to learn how you can achieve good health and wellness for life.

Unfortunately, too many people ignore their recommended preventive care visit, and we collectively are getting sicker, living fewer years, and spending an obscene amount of money on sick care.

Preventive care helps you manage your health risks

Everyone has health risks, and it is important that you understand yours. No one can avoid risk. However, there are many things you can do to reduce your risk. Think about it. Every time you get into a car, there is a risk of getting into an accident. You minimize your risks by wearing your seatbelt and following traffic lights, stop signs, and the speed limit. The same concept applies to your health.

Preventive healthcare can be compared to car maintenance, something most adults understand. You likely use the correct fuel, get regular oil changes and tune-ups, and buy insurance to cover accidents. This helps to ensure that your car doesn't break down on the freeway or develop issues that are cost-prohibitive to fix.

What you need to ask yourself is, "Are you willing to treat your body with the same consideration you treat your car?" If you wait to engage with a healthcare provider until you're so sick you can't ignore your symptoms, you may need more frequent (and more expensive) visits to your PCP and/or medical specialists for ongoing health management. In that case, you'll not only be looking at potentially crippling medical bills but also the possibility of a reduced quality of life and lost income from having to miss work. Chronic conditions that could have been prevented or managed early might limit your ability to enjoy daily activities, spend time with loved ones, or pursue your career goals. Furthermore, the stress of dealing with serious health issues can take a toll on your mental well-being and relationships.

If you are a woman or person of color, you have it a bit harder. You have more challenges and may face more discrimination in the healthcare system, and, as a result, may be at greater risk for chronic, often preventable, disease like heart disease, diabetes, and some cancers. But with the right knowledge and actions, you can take control of your health journey, be your best health advocate, and improve your outcomes.

Preventive care is cheaper than sick care

An annual preventive visit often does not have a co-pay and some insurance plans reward you for getting this visit, since it is cheaper for health insurers to keep you healthy than to pay for your healthcare when you become sick or need to be admitted to the hospital. If you are scheduled for an illness visit but are overdue for an annual preventive visit, your provider may be able to address both issues and bill under a preventive visit, saving you money and time. (Of course, if you only want your health problem addressed, that is your choice too!)

The truth about vaccines

Vaccines are a critical part of preventive healthcare. Since vaccines were introduced in the early 20th century, they were, without much debate, considered a good thing. They reduce the risk of being infected with viruses. Some viruses, like influenza (the flu) and COVID, mutate or change. This is why every year there is a new vaccine for these viruses. The vaccine may not necessarily prevent you from becoming sick, but if you do become sick, it will reduce the severity of your symptoms and help you recover more quickly.

During the COVID pandemic vaccines inappropriately became a hot button political issue. The reality is that we need vaccines, both in infancy and as we age. Some are critical when we are older adults.[3]

Billions of lives have been saved over the years through vaccines. Even with the COVID pandemic, millions more would have died without the vaccines. Smallpox is gone forever due to vaccines. Polio too—you rarely see polio in the developed world today. Chicken pox? Fewer children get chicken pox now because of the vaccine. Same with measles and mumps. Human papillomavirus (HPV) is the number one sexually transmitted infection (STI). If you've ever had sex, or are having sex, your chances of being exposed to HPV are high, even higher the more sexual partners you have had. The HPV vaccine is helping to reduce HPV-related illness and death.

Chapter Six

———

Whole Person Healthcare for Overall Wellness

My approach to health and wellness is whole person care because you don't exist in a bubble. Whole person care goes beyond physical symptoms, recognizing that your overall health and quality of life depend on maintaining good physical, mental, emotional, social, and spiritual well-being. These aspects of your health are deeply interconnected, each one influencing the others. Your environment, lifestyle choices, and personal history all play crucial roles in your overall wellness, affecting not only your present state but also your future health.

While your past influences your present health, it doesn't have to define your future well-being. As you seek to optimize your health, look for providers who promote whole person healthcare.

To illustrate the need for whole person care, I can offer a few examples of the danger of focusing on physical symptoms alone.

Example #1: the common cold

You may come in for a sick visit with a sore throat, cough, and congestion, demanding antibiotics because you want to get better quicker and get on with your busy life. This may be the first healthcare appointment you have had in years. You've had things to do, children to care for, bosses to please, long work hours so you can pay your bills or get that promotion, and stress caring for parents. Perhaps you don't have insurance or money to pay for visits or have never been told how important healthcare is.

Your healthcare provider, who knows little about you, asks about your symptoms—watery eyes, runny nose, sore throat, headache, shortness of breath, congestion, fever, chills, cough, if productive or not, the color of your mucous, etc. They ask when the symptoms started, what you've taken for them, whether you've had the same symptoms in the past. They may ask who you live with and if other people in your house have similar symptoms and if they were treated for anything? They should do a physical exam (but may not), which might include listening to your lungs and heart and looking into your eyes, ears, nose, and mouth. Based on your request for antibiotics, the provider may give you a prescription and send you on your way. Your medical chart may or may not have been reviewed with you (especially if your appointment was with a new provider or because you were only there for a cold).

But here's the thing. Colds are very common, often self-limiting, meaning they are caused by a virus, not bacteria. Some people are more prone to colds than others. Why? People who are chronically stressed (not eating well, sleep deprived, spend most of their days sitting, are in stressful jobs or living situations, or are lonely and isolated) may have immune systems that are weaker and cannot fend off the common cold.

A provider who offers whole person care and focuses on your overall wellbeing would discuss lifestyle as well as physical symptoms. They might prescribe comfort measures with you, like rest, hydration, over the counter pain relievers, nasal spray for congestion, or cough drops with menthol. They may explain why a quick fix now may affect your future health and lifestyle and use the visit to counsel you on ways to avoid future illness.

A provider who offers sick care may respond to your desire to get on with your life with a prescription for antibiotics, without testing to see if you have a bacterial infection. If you take antibiotics when you don't need them (antibiotics are only for bacterial infections, not viral infections), they may cause you more harm—if not now, later. In fact, the overuse of antibiotics for viral infections has caused a rapid increase in antibiotic resistance, a serious and growing health concern where bacteria develop the ability to defeat the drugs designed to kill them. Many antibiotics have already lost their effectiveness, so when you actually have a bacterial infection, they won't treat it.

Scientists have other concerns about antibiotic overuse as well. They are studying the effects of how antibiotics affect the gut microbiome—your digestive ecosystem. There is some concern that overuse of antibiotics could be associated with colorectal cancer.[4] Additionally, children who received multiple courses of antibiotics may experience early disruption in their developing gut microbiome and be at higher risk for health conditions later in life.

While antibiotics are crucial medicines for bacterial infections, they need to be used only when necessary and taken exactly as prescribed. You should never stop taking them for a bacterial infection before the full course is finished. Improper usage can lead to antibiotic resistance.

Example #2: yeast infection

Here is another example of how whole person care benefits your health—a very common one that I see regularly in my women's health practice. Maria made an appointment for vaginal itching. I'd never seen her before, but she was put on my schedule as a walk-in appointment. I read on her chart she had uncontrolled diabetes. Her chart showed she had many visits for the same issue and had been prescribed oral yeast medication five times over the past year. She also had tried over-the-counter yeast medication. But she never had an exam or had vaginal cultures taken to confirm that she had a yeast infection. She told me that the itching was so intense she could not sit and could not have sex with her husband, which was causing her more stress.

Because of her diabetes, I asked her about her diet. She told me her breakfast was sweet bread and coffee with milk and sugar. Sometimes she ate oatmeal. For lunch she normally ate a piece of meat with vegetables and three tortillas. For dinner, she had meat, rice, beans, and four tortillas.

Maria said she was taking her diabetes medication but that her doctor often "yelled at her" because she was not controlling her sugar. After criticizing her behavior, he gave her more medication. I asked if she had ever been told what she should eat and she replied that she was told, "to eat healthy." But her diet clearly demonstrated she did not understand what "healthy" meant. She was unaware that what she was eating was contributing to her uncontrolled diabetes. I asked her if she understood the relationship between what she ate and her recurrent yeast infections and she answered "no."

Physical symptoms are our bodies way of talking to us. For Maria, her body was trying to communicate with her via intense vaginal itching that she was not managing her diabetes. Her diabetes and yeast infection needed to be controlled not only by taking her medication but also by eating a low glucose diet (yeast loves to feast on sugar) and being more physically active. I could have given her a prescription and sent her on her way—the easy way out. Instead, I did an exam and found classic red and swollen labia with thick clumpy yellow-green discharge. I took a vaginal culture to make sure she had a specific type of yeast infection. I also checked for a urinary tract infection (UTI), because UTIs and yeast often present with similar complaints. The urine dipstick was negative (as was the urine culture that was sent to the lab).

I wrote a prescription and encouraged her to keep the area clean and dry, use an ointment-based moisture protectant like Vaseline during the day to sooth the area, and apply cold compresses for discomfort until the medication took effect. The vaginal culture came back positive for candida albicans (the most common type of yeast infection) and candida glabrata (the less common type). The medication I prescribed was appropriate for both types. When I followed up with her, she told me she felt better.

The point here is that she was never tested for yeast to begin with and was given medication that treated one type of infection but not the other, without having the conversation that her diet may be a contributing factor to her problem. Our visit provided an opportunity to discuss her diabetes, what was making it worse, and what could be done to make it better to prevent future yeast infections. Talking with her took some time, but I used our 20-minute visit well. She walked away with more knowledge than she had before.

These examples illustrate the fact there is more to your presenting problem than your symptoms. You cannot separate a health care (or in this case a sick care) issue from every other thing happening in your life. A healthcare provider with a whole person approach to care is more likely to uncover the root causes of your symptoms and understand how various aspects of your life interact to affect your health.

Chapter Seven

———

Where to Get the Healthcare You Need

Back when healthcare was simpler, if you had a health issue, you could call your doctor's office, speak to a familiar receptionist, and get clear guidance on what to do. Today, the landscape of healthcare has dramatically changed, making it less obvious where to seek care. With primary care offices, urgent care centers, retail clinics, telemedicine, and specialized facilities, the choices can be overwhelming.

In this chapter, I break down the different types of visits and what they typically involve, how they're billed, and what you can expect to pay as a patient. By understanding these distinctions, you'll be better equipped to choose the right type of care for your needs and understand the financial implications of your healthcare choices. Whether you're focusing on preventive care or dealing with an acute or chronic illness, this knowledge will help you navigate the healthcare system more confidently.

Wellness visit

The wellness visit, as noted earlier, is also known as an annual preventive health visit. It's generally done in a primary care office and involves a head-to-toe review of your body (asking you questions about any physical, mental, or emotional symptoms you may have) and your health history. This visit is more comprehensive than other types of visits. (See Chapter Nine for a complete rundown on this exam.) Your PCP will check your vital signs and prescribe blood work to screen for common illnesses like diabetes, heart disease, kidney or thyroid dysfunction and anemia. An annual preventive visit often does not have a co-pay and some insurance plans reward you for getting this visit.

Illness visit

When you have a specific problem, you make an appointment for an illness—or sick—visit. This appointment may be with your PCP or a medical specialist. Depending on your insurance, you may have a copayment for any illness visit. If you schedule an illness visit but are overdue for an annual preventive visit, your provider may be able to give you a checkup at the same time and bill for diagnosing and prescribing treatment for your illness under a preventive visit, saving you money and time.

Urgent care/immediate care visits

When you are ill and need to see a provider but can't get a same day appointment to see your own PCP (or you don't have a PCP), you can go to an urgent care/immediate care center in your area. Urgent and immediate care are different words for the same service. Urgent/immediate care clinics often have longer hours than primary care offices and may be open evenings and weekends. **Urgent care can be a cost-effective alternative to the emergency room for noncritical issues.** They may have more equipment than PCP offices but not as much as an emergency room. You can expect to pay higher copays for urgent care than a scheduled PCP visit, but that depends on your insurance coverage. The provider you see at urgent care will only address your urgent problem, not everything else happening in your body and life.

Retail clinics

Retail clinics, often found in pharmacies or big-box stores, offer convenient, walk-in care for common health issues like minor infections, vaccinations, and basic health screenings. They typically charge a flat fee for each service, which is often lower than traditional doctor's office visits. While these clinics provide quick access to care, they may not offer the continuity of care or comprehensive services that your PCP can. Complex health issues should still be addressed by your PCP or a specialist.

Emergency care

When you have a critical life-threatening issue, you should seek care in an emergency room/emergency department (ER/ED) at a hospital. (See the list below for what issues are considered critical and life-threatening.) In some remote areas, the ER may be the only place to get care. The ER is the only place that by law cannot turn you away and is open 24/7. However, because of its expense, emergency care should be avoided if your condition isn't critical. I see patients visit ERs for urinary tract infections, pregnancy tests, or sexually transmitted infection (STI) tests. Too often, patients seen in emergency departments are overtreated for potential infections even before their tests come back. For example, someone presenting with vaginal discharge or pelvic pain may be prescribed the antibiotics, doxycycline, ceftriaxone, and metronidazole. As I mentioned before, taking antibiotics when you don't have an infection can lead to more harm. You also don't get follow-up care when you go to the emergency room, even if you are a frequent flyer. Additionally, ER healthcare providers rarely have the time to educate you about health management when you have a chronic health condition like high blood pressure.

Important Note

Patient beware. Just because you can get emergency care does not mean that this care is free. It is the exact opposite. Emergency care is extremely expensive. Screenings such as a computed tomography (CT) scan that might cost under $500 when scheduled in advance can cost over $5,000 in the emergency room. You will be responsible for paying any portion of *the bill not covered by your insurance plan (or all of the bill if you don't have insurance). If you don't pay your bill, it will be sent to a Collections agency, which will affect your credit rating. In some cases, hospitals can offer financial aid (but may not bring it up). So, make sure you ask about this if you are uninsured, don't have Medicaid, or don't make enough money to pay off the full bill in your lifetime.*

Signs you need emergency care

The American College of Emergency Physicians provides the following tips for when to go to the emergency room. If your symptoms are not on the list, call your provider's office for guidance.

Keep in mind, this list does not represent every kind of sign or symptom that might occur, so if you think you or someone else may be having a medical emergency, call 911 or seek immediate medical care. When an emergency medical technician (EMT) comes to your house to check you out, they can determine if you need to go to the emergency department.

Adult Medical Emergency Symptoms

- Difficulty breathing, shortness of breath
- Chest or upper abdominal pain or pressure lasting two minutes or more
- Fainting[1], sudden dizziness, weakness
- Changes in vision
- Choking[2]
- Head or spine injury
- Injury due to a serious motor vehicle accident, burns or smoke inhalation, near drowning, deep or large wound or other serious injuries

---

1. https://www.emergencyphysicians.org/article/know-when-to-go/fainting

2. https://www.emergencyphysicians.org/article/health--safety-tips/choking--heimlich-manuever

- Ingestion of a poisonous substance
- Difficulty speaking
- Confusion or changes in mental status, unusual behavior, difficulty waking
- Any sudden or severe pain
- Uncontrolled bleeding[3]
- Severe or persistent vomiting or diarrhea
- Coughing or vomiting blood
- Suicidal or homicidal feelings
- Unusual abdominal pain[4]

Pediatric Medical Emergency Symptoms

- Severe headache or vomiting, especially following a head injury[5]
- Uncontrolled bleeding
- Inability to stand up or unsteady walking
- Unconsciousness
- Abnormal or difficult breathing
- Skin or lips that look blue or purple or gray
- Feeding or eating difficulties
- Increasing or severe, persistent pain
- Fever[6] accompanied by change in behavior (especially with a severe, sudden headache accompanied by mental changes, neck/back stiffness)
- Any significant change from normal behavior:
    - Confusion or delirium

3. https://www.redcross.org/take-a-class/first-aid/first-aid-training/first-aid-classes/until-help-arrives

4. https://www.emergencyphysicians.org/article/know-when-to-go/stomach-pain

5. https://www.emergencyphysicians.org/article/pediatrics/child-head-injury

6. https://www.emergencyphysicians.org/article/pediatrics/fever-in-children

48

- Decreasing responsiveness or alertness
- Excessive sleepiness
- Irritability
- Seizure[7]
- Strange or withdrawn behavior
- Lethargy

Anyone who thinks they're having a medical emergency should not hesitate to seek care. Federal law ensures that anyone who comes to the emergency department is treated and stabilized, and that their insurance provides coverage based on symptoms, not a final diagnosis. [5]

If English is not your first language

If you are not comfortable having a visit in English because it is not your preferred language, your provider does not speak your native language, or you are deaf and your provider doesn't sign, **by law in the USA, translation services need to be offered.** This is covered under the American with Disabilities Act.[6]

This is also true when making an appointment, registering for a visit, or interacting with anyone on your healthcare team. Of course, this makes common sense, but common sense is not so common. How are you going to get the most from your visit if the person caring for you does not understand you and you do not understand them? Some places have policies about having family members translate and this varies by clinic practice. Know that if you are not comfortable having a visit done solely in English because your provider does not speak your native language, it is your right to request a translator. The responsibility to find a translator is not yours nor should you ever be required to pay for translation services—it is the responsibility of the clinic/office.

---

7. https://www.emergencyphysicians.org/article/pediatrics/childhood-seizures

Patient's right to privacy

If you are bringing a child over 12 or an elderly parent or friend in for care, know that the patient has the right to privacy and should be asked if they wish to have their visit alone. Discuss this with the provider at the beginning of the visit. When a parent or guardian brings a teenager to see me, I always ask the patient if they want their parent there since I will be asking some sensitive, maybe embarrassing questions. I want them to feel free to be open and honest and develop trust in me. Most of the time, parents understand, but sometimes they get angry. I believe the sooner teenagers and young adults learn they have control over their own health—and learn how to be proactive—the more they will take responsibility for it as well.

Chapter Eight

———

Understanding Health Insurance

You probably buy insurance for your home or apartment, your car, and maybe even your phone so you can afford to replace these expensive essentials if they are damaged, lost, or stolen. However, when it comes to health insurance, you may think it's a luxury you can't afford. Health insurance is more important than any other kind of insurance. It's coverage for your body—the only one you'll ever have— and it ensures you're financially prepared for unexpected health issues.

No matter how healthy you are today, accidents and serious illnesses can happen to anyone, anytime. If you get really sick or hurt, it is human nature to want to go full force ahead with treatment recommendations that can cost tens of thousands, or even hundreds of thousands of dollars. The problem is no treatment is free. Emergency rooms have to treat and stabilize you, without asking for your insurance information; but they also will charge you. Medical bills can be financially devastating and our healthcare system is unforgiving when it comes to collecting the money they believe they are owed.

In 2023, 7.7% of the population, or almost 26 million Americans, were uninsured.[7] This is down from a high of 16% in 2010, but doesn't tell the whole story. In a 2022 study, 29% of people with employer health coverage and 44% of those with individual or publicly funded coverage were underinsured.[8] Healthcare debt is the number one cause of personal bankruptcy—and a major contributor to stress and anxiety.

My hope is that this chapter helps clarify the complex world of health insurance and explain your options so you get the insurance you need and never have to face the crippling agony of healthcare debt.

Who pays the bill?

Health insurance is one of our most hotly debated political topics. While most Americans agree that access to affordable care should be a human right, the U.S. is the only developed country that does not offer universal health care. Policy makers disagree on whether healthcare should be a shared or personal responsibility. Many believe the rich should not subsidize the poor. But I, like most Americans, believe that keeping everyone healthy benefits the community as a whole. Afterall, when people are healthy they can work more, have less sick time, fuel the economy, take care of their family and friends, and place less financial burden on our government sponsored healthcare plans.

Today, the U.S. healthcare system relies heavily on private insurance, with employers and/or individuals paying the premiums. Thanks to the Affordable Care Act (ACA), enacted in 2010, more individuals who don't have employer-sponsored benefits have access to affordable insurance through the publicly funded Marketplace or are covered by federally-sponsored programs including Medicare and Medicaid.

Employer-sponsored health insurance

Under the Affordable Care Act, employers with at least 50 full-time employees (those who work 30 hours or more a week) are required to offer affordable health insurance coverage to their full-time workers and their dependents up to age 26.

Corporations that compete for highly skilled workers and professionals may provide generous healthcare benefits, with no cost to the employee. However, health insurance benefits cut into company profits, so it's not uncommon for companies to offer health insurance with affordable premiums that have high deductibles and copays the average employee can't afford. Some companies may offer good benefits but lower their employees' salaries to cover their costs. Many companies with under 50 full-time employees do not offer benefits. Some companies limit their employees work to under 30 hours so that they don't have to offer any benefits.

The differences in employer-sponsored insurance coverage not only vary by the size and status of the company but also by the race and ethnicity of employees. Whites across the board are more likely to be insured by their employers while people of color have less access to jobs with good insurance benefits. Employers would have healthier workforces if they provided health insurance rather than consider their employees disposable and easily replaceable.

Individual health insurance market and public marketplaces

If you do not have health insurance benefits through your employer, you have the option of buying insurance directly from a private insurance company or through the public Health Insurance Exchange (Marketplace), developed through the Affordable Care Act (ACA). The ACA, originally known as Obamacare, gets a bad rap from many. But here's the thing. Healthcare insurance through a private insurance company is expensive. The ACA created an insurance marketplace for people who do not get health insurance through their employers, do not qualify for Medicaid, a state funded program, or live in a state that does not have expanded Medicaid. Every plan on the Marketplace has to meet specific standards, such as covering individuals with pre-existing conditions and providing essential coverage without an annual or lifetime benefit cap.

The Marketplace, which you can access through the website HealthCare.gov[1], provides subsidies that lower your premium costs if

1. https://www.healthcare.gov/

your household has an income between 100% and 400% of the federal poverty level. Each state is required to offer this insurance. In 2024, 18 states and Washington DC ran their own marketplaces, operating their own website platforms and customer service centers. Other states use the enrollment platform on the federal HealthCare.gov website.

The Marketplace makes health insurance incredibly affordable for the majority of Americans. The majority of people who qualify for subsidized insurance pay $10/month or less for premiums. But for those who are at higher income levels, premiums are higher. For those without a lot of disposable income or living paycheck to paycheck, the premiums can still seem high. To learn whether you qualify for subsidies and what your premium costs and benefits will be, visit Healthcare.gov.

Open enrollment for health insurance through the Marketplace is November 1 through January 15. If you have a life change or change in your employment or income, you may qualify for coverage during a special enrollment period.

As with employer funded health insurance plans, Marketplace plans, by law, must cover dependent children until the child reaches age 26.[9]

Publicly funded health insurance

Publicly funded health insurance includes Medicaid, Medicaid Expansion, Medicare, the Children's Health Insurance Program, Indian Health Service. With the exception of Medicare, which is run by a federal agency, publicly funded health insurance programs are administered by states and funded by both the federal and state governments. For three years during the pandemic, these programs were provided without the need to redetermine eligibility annually to ensure continuous coverage. When the pandemic-era policies ended in May 2023, many people suddenly lost their coverage because they didn't realize they now had to renew it. Many states expanded Medicaid coverage to help those people stay insured, whereas several states, particularly in the southeast have not, leaving the most vulnerable without coverage. Not surprisingly, the states with the poorest access to publicly funded health insurance have some of the poorest health outcomes.

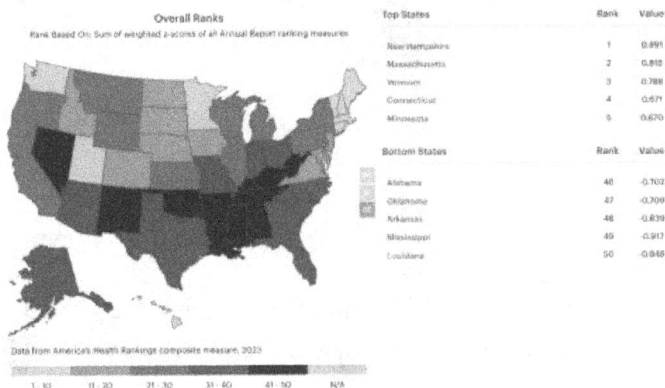

Overall by State
Rank based on: Sum of weighted z-scores of all Annual Report ranking measures

Source: America's Health Rankings United Health Foundation

https://www.americashealthrankings.org/api/v2/render/charts/ measure-national-summary/report/2023-annual-report/measure/ Overall/size/1200x600.png

or

56

Adult uninsured rates have fallen since 2019 but remain highest in states that have not expanded their Medicaid programs.

Percentage of adults ages 19-64 who are uninsured, by state (2021)

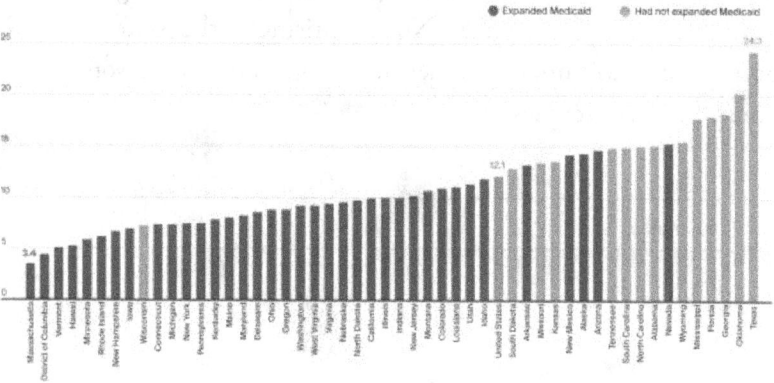

Note: States with orange shading had not fully expanded their Medicaid program under the Affordable Care Act by January 1, 2021.

Data: U.S. Census Bureau, 2021 One-Year American Community Survey, Public Use Microdata Sample (ACS PUMS).

Source: David C. Radley et al., *The Commonwealth Fund 2023 Scorecard on State Health System Performance: Americans' Health Declines and Access to Reproductive Care Shrinks, But States Have Options* (Commonwealth Fund, June 2023). https://doi.org/10.26099/rkgs-ud24

[↓] Download data

https://www.commonwealthfund.org/publications/scorecard/2023/jun/2023-scorecard-state-health-system-performance[2]

Medicaid is health insurance for low-income individuals and families, pregnant women, people with disabilities, and the elderly. Medicaid is mostly funded by the federal government, with states sharing a percentage of costs and the responsibility for determining who is eligible and how payments are made. Eligibility is based mostly on income but also other factors (each state has their own criteria). If you apply for health insurance through the public Marketplace, you will learn whether you qualify for Medicaid or should buy insurance through the Marketplace.

2. https://www.commonwealthfund.org/publications/scorecard/2023/jun/2023-scorecard-state-health-system-performance

Medicaid pays for clinic/office visits, prescriptions, maternity care, and behavioral health services. Medicaid also covers inpatient and home healthcare services. There may be other services provided as well, depending on the state you live in. You cannot use Medicaid from one state in another.

There are **straight Medicaid** plans where state governments pay directly for your healthcare services and **Managed Medicaid** plans that work with private insurance companies, who in turn pay for these services. Their fee structures are different but they both normally offer care coordination services within a network of eligible providers. If you are in a Managed Medicaid plan, you must receive services within a network of partners (specialists and hospitals and sometimes pharmacies). Not all healthcare providers accept Medicaid insurance (straight or managed) because those programs do not reimburse as much private insurance companies. Even if you're covered by a Medicaid health insurance plan, it may be more difficult to get care if the healthcare providers in your area do not accept it.

For more information about Medicaid in your state and to see if you are eligible check out the link in the resource section.

Medicaid Expansion is a program that lowers the requirements for individuals and families with incomes up to 138% of the poverty level to qualify for Medicaid. The federal government provides subsidies to states who have Expanded Medicaid programs, reducing costs to the states. States received additional financial incentives in the 2021 American Rescue Plan to expand Medicaid further. As of 2024, 40 states plus Washington D.C. had used the program to expand coverage, helping to reduce the racial inequities in healthcare.[10] While many states have also seen a reduction in their traditional Medicaid spending, many states continue to refuse expansion.

58

Status of State Action on the Medicaid Expansion Decision

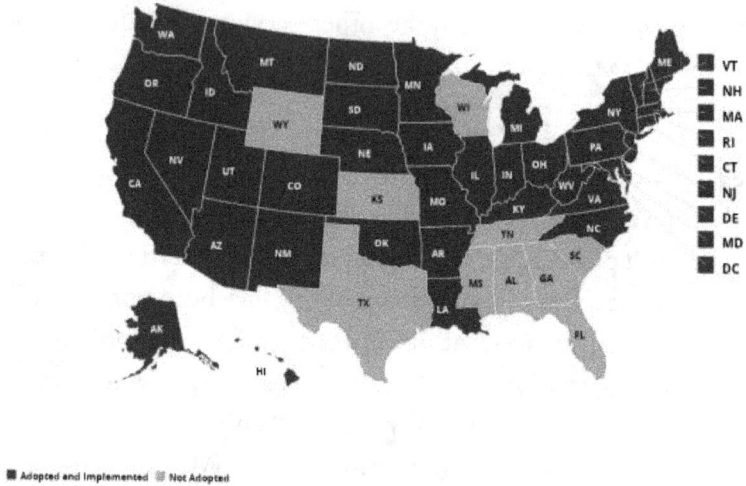

Adopted and Implemented Not Adopted

SOURCE: KFF kff.org

https://www.kff.org/medicaid/issue-brief/status-of-state-medicaid-expansion-decisions-interactive-map/[3]

In states that do not have expanded Medicaid, people whose incomes are below the federal poverty level do not qualify for Medicaid or the government subsidies to purchase reduced cost insurance on the Marketplace. They are at the mercy of community health centers. Without health insurance or the ability to afford healthcare, millions of people are at risk for chronic illness and early death. Voting for politicians who believe that healthcare is a right is one way you can improve everyone's chances of getting coverage and maintaining the coverage you have.

3. https://www.kff.org/medicaid/issue-brief/status-of-state-medicaid-expansion-decisions-interactive-map/

Medicare is a publicly funded health insurance plan for people 65 and older who are U.S. residents and either U.S. citizens or aliens with permanent residency status who've lived in the U.S. for 5 continuous years prior to applying for Medicare. Employees and the self-employed pay into the Medicare program through their taxes. Medicare is not income dependent. Some people with certain health conditions or disabilities can get Medicare without an age requirement. Medicare is a fully federally funded health insurance program.

For more information on all types of publicly funded health insurance, refer to the resources section at the end of this book.

The Children's Health Insurance Program (CHIP) is a health insurance program available in every state for children ages 0 to 19 whose family incomes do not qualify for Medicaid. The insurance is not free, but the charge is minimal based on income.

All children receiving Medicaid—either straight, Medicaid Managed or CHIP—often lose coverage at age 19, at which point they need to apply for their own insurance through Medicaid, the Marketplace, or an employer.

Indian Health Service is a federally funded program providing comprehensive health services to American Indians and Native Alaskans.

The ABCDs of Medicare: The Original Medicare and Medicare Advantage

Last I checked, over 40% of seniors live on Social Security alone.[11] Some may receive pensions from their employers, though this is rarer today than it was a few decades ago. Social Security Insurance is barely enough to live on let alone use to pay for healthcare related expenses. Fortunately, Americans have access to federally supported Medicare coverage when they hit 65. But that doesn't mean you'll be free from all medical expenses. It's more critical than ever to take good care of yourself when you're younger so you can reduce your healthcare expenses as you get older.

If you are approaching Medicare age, have recently become eligible for Medicare, or dislike the plan you have, **it helps to have a good understanding of how the program works.** There are different plans and ways to take advantage of Medicare coverage.

Original Medicare

Original Medicare includes three parts:

Part A is hospital insurance that covers inpatient, skilled nursing, nursing home, hospice and some home health care. It does not cover preventive exams or dental and vision care. This coverage is available with no additional charge to the individual.

Part B is medical insurance that covers two types of services: preventive health care and medically necessary services. There is a monthly premium for Part B in addition to an annual deductible ($240 in 2024) and a 20% co-pay of the total amount Medicare approves for each service. There is no yearly limit on your maximum out-of-pocket expenses per year. (See below for information on supplemental insurance coverage (Medigap) or Medicaid you can add to your plan to help pay your 20% co-insurance.)

Part D is Medicare drug coverage. Medicare's website states "Even if you don't take prescription drugs now, consider getting Medicare drug coverage. If you decide not to get it when you're first eligible, and you don't have other creditable prescription drug coverage (like drug coverage from an employer or union) or get Extra Help, you'll likely pay a late enrollment penalty[4] if you join a plan later. Generally, you'll pay this penalty for as long as you have Medicare drug coverage."[12] (Extra Help is a program that helps cover deductibles and copays for prescription drugs for limited income individuals.)

When you accept Original Medicare, you can use any provider or hospital that takes Medicare anywhere in the U.S. You do not need a referral to see a specialist.

Part C Medicare Advantage

Part C, also known as Medicare Advantage, is coverage you buy from private insurance companies that combines Part A, Part B, and often Part D into one Medicare-approved plan. When you elect to have a Medicare Advantage plan, you pay the private insurance company a monthly premium (often quite low) and don't pay Medicare Part B. Medicare Advantage plans often offer benefits like vision, hearing, and dental coverage that aren't included in Original Medicare.

Most Medicare Advantage plans only cover providers in a specific network, normally where you live, and don't cover non-emergency out-of-state care. Some plans offer state-to-state coverage, but these plans generally are more expensive. You may need a referral from your PCP to see a specialist. Your maximum annual out-of-pocket costs may be less than with Original Medicare, but co-pays and deductible can vary from plan to plan. **It's important to compare plans and look carefully at what the plans cover and what your deductible and copays will be.**

Since these plans are run by private healthcare organizations that are given a set amount of money from Medicare each year based on the number of patients covered, the theory is that the organizations will work hard to ensure their patient base stays healthy and does not need

4. https://www.medicare.gov/drug-coverage-part-d/costs-for-medicare-drug-coverage/part-d-late-enrollment-penalty

avoidable and unnecessary medical services and hospitalizations. Unfortunately, some of these organizations have not done well at keeping patients healthy and increase their profits by denying patients coverage for various medical services. Before choosing a Medicare Advantage program, talk to friends who may have a plan and check reviews online to determine the reputation of the organization.

Medicare Supplement Insurance

Medicare Supplement insurance, also called Medigap, is insurance you can add to Original Medicare after you've signed up for Medicare Part A and Part B. It helps cover the 20% copays and any co-insurance and deductibles that aren't covered by Medicare, which can get quite high if you require a lot of health care.

There are 10 different types of Medigap plans offering different benefit levels. These types have letter names, starting with Plan A and ending with Plan N. No matter what insurance company you buy your policy from, each plan is standardized and offers the same basic benefits. Plan A for instance covers coinsurance and copayments not covered by Medicare Part A and Part B whereas Plan G covers all that as well as deductibles, excess charges, skilled nursing facility coinsurance, and 80% of foreign travel emergency. Some plans have no out-of-pocket limit while others limit coverage to 50% of your out-of-pocket costs until you meet your out-of-pocket annual limit.

The only difference between Medigap policies is the price of the premium you pay. Certain companies may offer additional benefits, such as gym memberships and online health apps. Most will give you the option of buying additional coverage for dental, vision, and hearing.

Understanding your coverage

Health insurance, like other insurance, must be renewed every year and every year the terms and conditions (and cost) may change. There is an open enrollment period to sign up for health insurance, whether you're getting it from your employer, the state, or through the federal health insurance Marketplace. That enrollment period may vary from state to state or company to company.

Before you sign up for any insurance plan, you must be given access to information that tells you what and what is not covered and what the policy will cost you. You can research your options online on the Marketplace, Managed Medicaid, or Medicare Advantage plan websites before you sign on the dotted line and commit yourself for one year. Most employers should also give you online access to your health insurance options.

Once you enroll in a policy, the insurer must send you a printed packet of information for reference. If you are going to lose coverage or your coverage is going to change, you must also be informed in writing. It may seem tedious to read through the details, but being informed about your benefits and coverage can save you headache, heartache and money in the long run.

When evaluating plans, you will generally have the choice of a Health Maintenance Organization (HMO) or a Preferred Provider Organization (PPO). Both are alike in that they include a network of healthcare providers to choose from. But they have some significant differences:

An HMO is the most affordable health insurance plan with lower monthly premium payments and lower out of pocket expenses (deductible). It covers healthcare services provided within a designated network of primary care providers, specialists, hospitals, and radiology services. When you select an HMO plan, you are limited by where you can receive care. You must pick a Primary Care Provider (PCP) that is part of this network and get a referral (order) from your provider to see a specialist. If you see a provider out of network, your insurance company may pay only part of or none of the bill. This may include emergency rooms.

A PPO is the most flexible healthcare insurance plan, but it is also the most expensive. Premiums are higher but you generally get to select care from a much larger network of providers (outpatient or inpatient). The plan covers both in-network and out-of-network providers, generally without needing a referral. However, your co-pays and co-insurance are generally lower if you see an in-network provider.

To help you compare health insurance plans, here are the most common features you'll be evaluating. This list is not exhaustive.

Premium:

The amount of money you pay each month for your insurance. If you get it from an employer, it will be taken out of your paycheck. If you have Original Medicare and get Social Security benefits, it will be deducted from your monthly Social Security payment. Typically, the cost for employer provided health insurance is divided by you and your employer. You will see a deduction for your health insurance on each paystub. The amount of the premium depends on what type of insurance plan you choose (PPO, HMO) and how many people are being insured on your insurance plan (if you are insuring yourself, you will pay less than if you are insuring your spouse and/or children).

Deductible:

Is the out-of-pocket expense you pay for some health services and medications before your health insurer pays. If you have a deductible of $1500, then your insurance will not pay for services until you have met this deductible. Most preventive services are paid in full, whether or not you've met your deductible. This is another reason to prevent illness from occurring in the first place!

Some insurance plans offer a high deductible option (say $10,000). This may seem appealing because your monthly premium payment is lower, BUT if you have a major healthcare event, you are stuck having to pay all out-of-pocket costs up front until you meet that $10,000 deductible and your insurance coverage kicks in. In some cases, if you can afford to, it may make sense to go with the higher deductible and put the money you would have spent on higher premiums into a savings account. Then, you can use your savings to pay medical bills until insurance starts covering them. If you don't use medical services that year, you'll have savings you can use for future medical bills.

Co-payments:

This is a fixed amount you pay for services. You may find your co-payment (co-pay) amount on your insurance card. There are co-pays for illness visits, specialists, emergency room or urgent/immediate care visits. In-network co-pays are lower than out of network co-pays. Annual preventive and family planning visits do not (should not) have co-pays nor should screenings like mammograms and colonoscopies.

You may also have co-payments (co-pays) for your prescription medication, higher co-pay for branded medication, lower for generic. Your co-pay may be lower if you opt for mail order medication, a three-month supply rather than a 30-day supply. Birth control should not have a co-pay however, many are uninformed and are still paying for contraception. The New York Times published an article June 26, 2024 "Contraception is Free by Law. So Why Are a Quarter of Women Still Paying for It? https://www.nytimes.com/2024/06/26/birth-control-pills-contraception-cost.html

Knowledge is power and the more you know about what your insurance covers and what is the cost to you, the better. The more you know, the more motivated I hope you will be to take control of your health and wellness to avoid financial pitfalls.

Co-insurance:

Co-insurance is the percentage of the total costs you pay. Unlike co-pays that have a fixed amount, your co-insurance percentage is based on the total bill for services. Your co-insurance may be 20%, meaning you pay 20% of the allowed amount your insurance company will pay for a particular service. If you had a provider visit that was $200, you would be responsible for $40 plus the set co-pay, if you have one. Your co-insurance cost will depend on whether you have met your deductible. Once you've met it, you no longer have to pay co-pays or co-insurance.

HSA: Health Savings Account

Some health insurance plans let you set aside a Health Savings Account. If you have a high deductible plan, a health savings account deducts money from your paycheck before taxes, and you can use the money to help pay for health-related expenses like deductibles, co-insurance, vision, dental and other healthcare related expenses. The unused money in your HSA rolls over to the next year. The money you select to put in your HSA is not taxable.

If you cannot qualify for any government funded health insurance plan

If you do not have health insurance, cannot afford to purchase insurance through the Marketplace (not even catastrophic insurance if you are under 30) and do not qualify for Medicaid, look for Federally Qualified Health Centers (FQHC) in your area. I will provide a link in the resources section where you can find an FQHC. FQHCs provide healthcare based on a sliding fee—meaning your cost is based on what you earn and your family size. The price you pay includes the visit and lab work, but not medications. However, FQHCs often have agreement with pharmacies where patients can get discounted medication pricing under the 340B program (it's complicated, but helpful to know it exists). All FQHCs offer primary care (pediatrics, family medicine and women's health) but some also offer behavioral health and dental care too for an affordable cost.

If you have no health insurance but were given a medication prescription by a PCP, urgent/immediate care clinic, or emergency room provider, there are affordable ways to purchase medications. See the resources section for options.

Chapter Nine

———

Anatomy of a Primary Care Visit

Now that you have an idea of who you can see and where to see them, I'm going to walk you through a good visit, and give you the tools you need to be an active participant in your own care. You may be thinking, this is not my job, my provider should be doing everything for me. I get that, but for the patient-provider relationship to be good—and for you to get the care you deserve—you and your providers need to work together.

If your provider isn't responsive, you may have the choice to change providers. Unfortunately, there are "healthcare deserts" where your options are limited. A provider shortage, combined with health insurance plans that restrict where you can get care, make it harder to switch providers and crucial to maximize each visit you have. You want to get everything you need from that interaction, since your next opportunity may be far off. Advocating for yourself doesn't always get you the best care, but it should improve the care you get.

Step one: preparation for your visit

If you are an established patient to your PCP's office, you have access (or should be given access) to your electronic medical record (EMR) via a patient portal, MyChart, or other online app. EMRs have been around for over a decade and provide a centralized, easily accessible, and comprehensive view of a patient's health history. They are designed to make it easier for providers to improve care coordination, reduce medical errors, and communicate more efficiently with other healthcare providers across different settings. Hopefully your provider is not still writing everything down in a paper chart.

If you have no idea what I am talking about, The ONC Cures Act Final rule[1] states that all patients must be given access to their medical record.[13] You read that right—**it is the law that you are given access to your medical record**. Your patient portal allows you to track upcoming health services, helping you stay on top of preventive care and routine check-ups for better overall health management. Depending on your age and sex, these services may include a pap smear, mammogram, prostate exam, colon cancer screening, skin cancer screening, vaccines, certain labs if you have chronic health conditions like diabetes or high blood pressure, and upcoming routine visits. By reviewing this information before your appointment, you can prepare questions and potentially schedule multiple services for the same visit.

Step two: early arrival

When you make your appointment, you may be instructed to arrive early, either on your patient portal, in a text sent to you before your visit, or a telephone call from the office. This allows extra time to complete any necessary paperwork, verify current insurance, and pay your co-pay before your actual appointment with the provider. Your provider most likely has a booked schedule. So, if you arrive ten minutes late and your appointment was only booked for 20 minutes, you may not be seen, since that may back up all other appointments for the rest of the day. On the flip side, your PCP should also be ready to see you at the appointed time, which doesn't always happen. Providers frequently run behind schedule due to overbooking and insufficient time between appointments. They generally won't—and shouldn't— dismiss patients who have more questions or complex health issues to address than their allotted times allowed for.

---

1. https://www.healthit.gov/sites/default/files/page2/2020-03/TheONCCuresActFinalRule.pdf

Many PCPs, in fact, are leaving the profession because they are frustrated by not having control over their schedules. These PCPs work as employees of large healthcare organizations and are limited by what their employers tell them they have to do (such as not giving patients as much time as they'd like to). While this is not your problem, it's important to understand why you may not be seen on time, so you don't blame your provider for the wait.

Important Note:

If you make an appointment and do not show up, this prevents another patient from being seen (remember you probably waited a long time to see your provider, as are other patients). Some practices have a policy and charge you when you do not keep an appointment, while other practices, especially ones that accept Medicaid, cannot charge you when you do not show. Someone must be accountable and at the end of the day, your provider gets pressured for not seeing enough patients.

Step three: health and lifestyle questionnaire

After checking in for your appointment, a medical assistant or nurse will greet you and bring you to the examining room. They will ask you your name and date of birth (to make sure they are taking care of the correct person). They will ask you the reason for your visit. This is called the chief complaint. You will be asked a series of questions to screen for intimate partner/domestic violence, depression, and anxiety. They will also ask whether are you having difficulty paying for necessities like rent/mortgage, utilities, bills, food, and medical care. (In some cases, you may be given a questionnaire to fill out instead of being asked these questions in person.)

Why are these questions asked? Whole person healthcare requires that we consider not just your physical health but anything that affects it. You are more than your chief complaint. Everything that happens in your world—at home, at work, in your relationships, where you live, what you eat, drink, how much you sleep and move, has an impact on your health and why you made the appointment. If you cannot meet your basic needs, your physical and mental health is affected. This can affect your health, today, tomorrow and in the future.

In healthcare, the term "social determinants of health" describes circumstances happening in your life that directly or indirectly affect health. Social determinants can affect anyone but are most associated with under-resourced inner city and rural communities. Concerns about finances, housing, employment, access to food, food costs, paying back student loans, credit card and other debt, access to health care (waiting months to get a healthcare provider appointment), poor quality healthcare, loneliness, and isolation are all too common and should not be hidden from your healthcare provider.

If you struggle with any lifestyle issues, you should be given resources to help improve your situation. I know that not all resources will be available in all areas. For example, affordable housing is a big problem that a healthcare provider has limited resources to solve. But knowing that you have unstable housing or stress about finances should clue your provider into how difficult it may be for you to meet your health goals.

You should also be asked if you have seen another care provider or been seen in the emergency room since your last visit, whether you have any allergies to medications, and what medications are you taking. You may also be asked by the medical assistant or nurse if you are smoking cigarettes, vaping, or using smokeless tobacco products.

Important Note

A note about financial literacy. The trend to use installment payments to buy clothing, shoes, and any consumer good has landed people in debt. Many people have not created budgets for themselves and live off credit cards and take out loans to buy homes, cars, and education with high interest rates. They lack the knowledge to compute how long it will take to pay the loans back. The higher the debt and the longer you have it hanging over you, the more stress you'll feel. The government offers online resources[2] to help you understand financial literacy.[14]

Step four: your vital signs

The medical assistant or nurse will take your vital signs, including height, weight, blood pressure, pulse, respirations, maybe oxygen saturation, temperature and, if you're female, ask for the first day of your last menstrual period (LMP). Sometimes, you may be asked to rate your pain on a 10-point scale (0 = no pain, 10 = the worst pain of your life).

Why is this information important? Because comparing your readings to a normal scale gives you and your provider a better understanding of your health or illness state. Imagine your health visit as a painting. The artist begins with an outline (your vital signs) and fills in the outline with color (your health history and physical exam) before placing the final touches (your healthcare plan). This will make more sense as you read on.

Step five: review of medications

You will be asked what medications you are taking (often, you are asked to bring all medications, vitamins, and supplements you take with you to your visit). Your list of medications and supplements will be reviewed with you by the medical assistant or nurse and then again by your provider. This is because multiple providers may have prescribed different medications without being aware of everything

2. *https://www.occ.gov/topics/consumers-and-communities/community-affairs/resource-directories/ financial-literacy/index-financial-literacy-resource-directory.html*

you take. When they are all listed in your EMR, it helps avoid medication errors or overprescribing.

Since not all medical offices, clinics, and hospitals use the same EMR system and not all EMR systems talk with each other, your primary care provider's list may not be complete. This is a good reason why it is important for your provider to ask you if you have been seen elsewhere, what medications have been prescribed and why, and which ones you are taking now. Your medication list should only include current medications. Bad things can happen if some medications are mixed or over prescribed. This has become a critical issue in providing quality care. Due to the opioid crisis, controlled substances with a high potential for addiction or misuse are now tracked in a national database. This system helps prevent overtreating you with certain medications and reduces the risk of you obtaining multiple prescriptions from different providers.

Step six: meeting with PCP

Before your provider comes in, the medical assistant or nurse may instruct you to undress and put on a gown. Regardless of the reason for your visit, I recommend that you **never begin your appointment with your healthcare provider undressed**, especially if you have never met them before. Even if you know you need a breast check, pap smear, pelvic exam, or prostate exam, wait to get undressed until after they have reviewed your medical record. If you need to have a breast or pelvic exam, you should always be asked if you want a chaperone in the room, even with a female provider. This is asked for your comfort level.

You feel more vulnerable—especially if you don't know the provider or have experienced prior trauma—when you are hiding behind a paper gown and the other person is fully clothed. In most cases, when you start the visit with your clothes on, you can lower the power dynamic and be on a more equal footing when you discuss your health concerns.

You can wait to undress for any necessary screenings until after your provider has spoken with you. While putting on the paper gown before they enter the room saves your PCP time, if you need to get undressed for a screening, it only takes a few minutes. Your PCP can walk out of the room and take a 2-minute break while you get ready. Of course, if you have been seeing your provider for a long time and are comfortable getting undressed in advance, then go ahead.

Step seven: medical record review

While your PCP may handle the first five steps of your appointment themselves, most larger clinics want their providers to focus their limited time with patients on diagnosis and treatment decision making.

It is standard practice for your provider to review your medical record at least once each year before seeing you, especially if you are a new patient. They should then review it again with you during the visit, even if you have previously been seen by this or other providers in the practice. This is to ensure that someone is updating your health history and your chart is kept current. Your health history can be updated with information from other healthcare systems, including medications, problem lists, and immunizations. This is possible when systems have compatible electronic medical records (EMRs). Your provider can simply click a button to access this information. In Epic, the EMR my organization uses, there are two icons I can choose. One tells me what new medications a patient has been prescribed and gives me a problem list and immunizations. The other is a list of all organizations that have compatible EMRs so I can read visit notes, see lab results, and other tests that were done.

Anything related to your health that has happened since your last visit should be added to your chart. For example, if you were in urgent care or the emergency department for an infection, car accident, or a fall, even if you weren't diagnosed with any major injuries, months later you could develop residual pain or other complications. If your PCP can see you had the illness or accident, they can then consider that as a possible cause for your current complaint or at the very least, something that is contributing to your pain.

Truth be told, whether a provider is seeing you for the first time or it has been a long time since your last visit, if they don't review your chart with you, it's a sign they don't care enough about you.

Your medical record is your life's novel and all progress notes over the years are chapters of your story. Any health professional should be able to read through your chart and know your health and wellness status, your current health problems if you have any, and the plan for managing your health and wellness. This should make it easier to quickly update your chart at future visits.

Personally, I like to review charts with patients, I can start a conversation where they ask me questions and I provide education. As I'm updating the chart, I can develop trust with new patients and catch up with established patients. I like to compare coming to see me with going to a buffet. I highlight what tests and screenings are recommended, what is due, explain the reasoning and rationale, and offer you treatment options, if needed, without pressure. You get to decide what you want from this buffet. It's your body, your health, your choice. Your time is just as valuable as mine.

If a patient is well known to me and it has been months since their last visit, I will ask if anything has changed in their or their family's history since their last visit. This gives me the opportunity to deepen my relationship with my patients. I laugh and cry with my patients. I am open and honest when I need to be, to demonstrate my understanding of what they are going through.

While healthcare providers are living life just like you, many feel they cannot admit it. Many providers think being vulnerable with patients is a taboo. They feel they must hold this power over their patients because they are the experts. I disagree. We are human just like you. We are patients too. We are not superheroes. We may be living with the same illnesses and life struggles.

If you feel like you're getting the cold shoulder from your provider, it can help the relationship to ask them if they have ever experienced anything like what you're dealing with. Showing my vulnerabilities and humanness with patients when it is appropriate has allowed me to build stronger and more trusting relationships. The greatest gift I have been given in my career is that women have trusted me with their vulnerabilities, have let me into their lives and shared with me their pains and joys, letting me support them in any way I can. Sometimes the support is to just listen and validate their concerns. I have learned so much from them and I am the provider today because of them.

Step eight: your health screenings

Your PCP will outline what screenings you're due to have (i.e. blood tests, mammograms, pap smears, colonoscopies, prostate exams) and any treatment options they think will support your health. You get to choose whether you want to follow their recommendations. You might be ready and willing or you may need time to consider your options.

I've found that when it comes to screenings, vaccinations, and prescription medication, some patients are scared to consider them. With screenings, it may feel better to not know than get unwelcome results. I see this a lot when it comes to mammograms. Patients may have heard they are painful or have family members who've had breast cancer and don't want to know if they have it too.

If you have concerns about any of the tests that are recommended, it may put you at ease to have a conversation with your PCP, explaining why you're worried and letting them explain why a test or procedure is recommended. If it doesn't help you, you have the right to refuse. That is ok.

I have cried with many patients over their risk factors and their refusal not to take my advice and recommendations. Some patients refuse to return to me because they don't want me to try to change their mind. Does it turn into preaching? Pleading? Probably. Have I ever felt like a failure when unable to persuade a patient to adopt healthier lifestyle choices or take medication to reduce their risk of surrendering to the same fate as a family member? Yes. More times than I want to count. But I have to respect their decision. Your body. Your choice. Your health.

Step nine: assessment and treatment plan

After collecting information by talking with you, doing a physical exam, and reviewing your health screening results, your PCP will make an assessment. If you have made the appointment due to an illness, they will make a diagnosis or several diagnoses.

After the assessment or diagnoses, your provider will make a care plan and go over it with you to make sure you understand next steps.

Medications

If you were prescribed medications, make sure they are sent to the correct pharmacy (you should have been asked for your preferred pharmacy at the very beginning of your visit). Also, make sure you understand how and when you are to take the medication. If you are being prescribed a new medication, ask about the side effects and medication alternatives so you are not caught off guard.

Two reasons why people stop taking their medication or do not take them as prescribed: price and side effects. Discuss costs with your PCP (name brands are not necessarily better than generic, but the cost differences vary widely). See if you have time to check and see what your insurance co-pay will be (even many Medicaid and Medicare plans have a co-pay to reduce their costs). Ask if taking two pills rather than one that combines medication may be more affordable. Some medications need to be taken with food, some can cause skin sensitivity to the sun and you will need to wear sunscreen. (You should be wearing sunscreen anyway.) Some medications can leave a metallic taste in your mouth or cause a cough. Will any of these be reasons you can't take that medication?

Medications are typically prescribed to be taken once a day, twice a day (or every 12 hours); three times a day (or every 8 hours while awake), four times per day (or every 6 hours while awake) or as needed. When you pick up the medications and you have questions, be sure to ask the pharmacist.

Referrals

A referral is an order to see someone else, usually a specialist. Sometimes healthcare providers do not have all the answers, and your presenting complaint may baffle us. We may turn to Dr. Google, Dr. Bing, Dr. Duck Duck Go, Up to Date and other resources to help us help you. But not every provider will admit they aren't sure what you're dealing with or what is causing it. We may order more tests or refer you to medical specialists, leaving you feeling frustrated.

Americans have become impatient in practically all aspects of our lives. Healthcare is no different, and I would argue there is even more impatience in healthcare. You want answers and you want them now. But the human body can be a mystery, and sometimes we need time and tests to figure it out, which can be worrisome. I understand. A good provider will admit when they do not have the answers and will explain the need for tests or referrals to a specialist and give you a sense of when you can expect answers.

There are specialists for everything. For instance, just for your head there is an ENT specialist for your ears, nose, and throat; an ophthalmologist who specifically evaluates your eyes; a neurologist who focuses on your brain; and a dermatologist who evaluates your skin.

We have divided the human body into so many parts, but last I checked, the human body is one complete whole. The healthcare system does not treat the human body as a complete whole—mind and body working together. Whether due to comfort level, burnout, or because there is so much more information to learn about human anatomy, we have created a system of specialists. And many PCPs find it easier to send a patient to a specialist rather than care for the patient themselves. Not all PCPs will consider whether they can manage the condition themselves. Many won't care about how long their patient will have to wait to see a specialist.

There are cases where a referral is definitely needed, such as to have specific studies like an ultrasound, x-ray, mammogram or colonoscopy. These can generally not be done at your provider's office. If you are not sure why you need a referral, ask. There needs to be a diagnosis for the referral to be made. Your provider cannot order something without relating it to a symptom or physical exam finding. Without that, your insurance company will not pay.

Also ask if your PCP or their support team can tell you what specialists your insurance company will pay for. (You may want to check your insurance coverage before your appointment to see what labs, imaging centers, and healthcare networks are included on your plan.) This may seem like too much work. Let me tell you as a provider, it is frustrating to have to recreate referrals when insurance companies reject them. It is also more frustrating for you to return for a new referral, especially if something concerning was detected and you want it diagnosed quickly. If it took you a long time to get an appointment to see your provider, it may take you even longer to see a specialist or get an ultrasound or mammogram. It is better to know where you can go so you get the services you need ASAP and won't be charged an out-of-pocket fee.

Step ten: progress notes

All providers should write progress notes based on their examination of you. Sometimes they do this while talking with you and sometimes they complete their notes after you've left. Their progress notes are based on a SOAP note format:

- **S = Subjective.** This is information you provide. It covers your history—medical, family, social, and surgical. It covers the reason for your visit—your chief complaint, when it started, if you've had the same issue before, what treatments you've had for it, and other symptoms. It may also include issues related to other organ systems in your body. If you're having an annual exam, there may be more details included in the progress notes for this visit.

- **O = Objective.** Think of this information as data. Your vital signs, your physical exam findings, and blood work results from previous visits. This information is fact and cannot be changed.

- **A = Assessment.** The diagnosis/diagnoses your provider came up with during your visit. It may be something very specific or something vague because they still need to find out the cause of a problem. Connected to these diagnoses will be anything ordered for those specific diagnoses like blood work, medication, referral to a specialist or for counseling, and the treatment options discussed with you.

- **P = Plan.** What is your care plan? This includes whatever was discussed at your visit, what education was provided, and what the plan is for follow-up or for your next appointment.

Basically, everything that occurred during your visit is summarized in the progress note. You should always have access to your progress notes in the patient portal. In the following two chapters, I break this down into more detail so you understand what should be in your chart.

Step eleven: after visit summary/discharge papers

Before you leave, if you have the option, look over your visit summary. You should be able to review your vital signs (weight, blood pressure, pulse), visit assessments (diagnoses), whatever medications were ordered or discontinued from your medication list, labs that were ordered, and any important instructions or education you were given by your provider during your visit. If you aren't given a paper copy, you should be given instructions on how you can sign up for the patient portal to review your EMR online and review your visit summary as well as get your test results.

Look over your referrals carefully. You will probably need to call to schedule your appointments. If you need assistance, especially if you do not speak English well, ask someone in your PCP's office to help you. You do not want to delay care because you are unfamiliar with the referral process. If you were told you needed a follow-up appointment, make sure it has been scheduled (especially if the wait time to get an appointment with your PCP is long).

Your goal is to leave your visit with all your questions answered. When in doubt ask. If your provider gets frustrated with you—tough! You made the appointment for YOU!

Chapter Ten

———

Your Health History: Subjective Information

Your health history, the subjective part of your medical record, is composed of many parts: medical, surgical, family, and social—your past and your present. It's important that you keep it as updated as possible. Anytime something changes in any part of your health history, it should be entered into your electronic medical record (EMR). Your EMR also has a problem list—a summary of your current health status—and this should reflect your current chronic health problems. You can review your EMR online and may be able to update all or parts of your health history, including medical, surgical, family, obstetric and social before your visit. If not, your PCP needs to transfer the answers in the questionnaire you filled out into your EMR to make sure this information has been included and is kept updated. This is an opportunity for your PCP to get to know you and your health history better and for you to get to know and develop trust in them.

Unfortunately, not all health systems and provider offices use the same technology for their electronic health records. The industry is working on interoperability—a big word for sharing information between providers who use different electronic health record systems. While the goal is to have every provider in the US able to see every other healthcare provider or emergency department you've visited, the lab tests and screenings you've had, and what medications and treatments you've been prescribed, not all systems can talk with each other. Urgent care center visit information, even when visible, is usually limited to prescribed medication. Additionally, you need to sign a consent form for sensitive information, such as abortions or mental health treatment, for those issues to be included on shared records.

Epic and Cerner are two of the largest electronic health record systems in the country. Patients treated in healthcare systems using these software platforms often find it easier to see all pieces of their healthcare puzzle, especially if they've received care in multiple locations. Since my practice uses Epic, sometimes I surprise patients by mentioning a recent hospital visit or medication they've had. When they wonder how I know these details, I can show them exactly where this information appears in their EMR. The level of detail available depends on how advanced the electronic health record system is.

In my clinic, for instance, during an annual wellness visit, I can open a "Labs" tab to view recent lab results and whether they were done at our clinic or elsewhere. This integration allows me to avoid repeating a test unnecessarily if labs are normal or if it's not yet time for a recheck. This is also true for diagnostic tests like ultrasounds or x-rays. This streamlined access to information helps me provide more efficient, coordinated, and cost-effective care.

The reality is, not all providers check through the EMR, often reordering screenings or lab tests you've already had. If the insurance company declines to approve that reordered test, you may be responsible for paying the bill. **If you think you've had a similar test done recently, question the provider about why it's necessary to have it done again.**

Your medical history

Your medical history began the day you were born and ends the day you die. You may not think that things in your past are relevant to your health (truth be told, you may not want to remember negative or traumatic experiences). **Just like anything you do now will affect your life today and into the future (hopefully well into your 80s), your past also impacts your current state of health.**

For instance, childhood illnesses can impact your health as an adult. If you ever had chicken pox, you are at risk for developing shingles. Rheumatic fever as a child can affect your heart health. If you have ever been pregnant and experienced complications during or after your pregnancy, like gestational diabetes or preeclampsia, this increases your risk for type 2 diabetes and hypertension. Any prior medical conditions are important for your healthcare provider to know.

Your medical history includes issues related to anemia, blood transfusions, anxiety, depression, abuse, trauma, diabetes, high blood pressure (hypertension), heart disease, and problems with your ears, eyes, nose, liver, lungs, kidneys, bones, and muscles. Basically, it includes any part or system of your body. Your medical history also includes hospitalizations and medical procedures you have had during your life.

There may be parts of your medical history you don't want to disclose, especially if it involves trauma, abuse, or neglect. That is ok. **It takes time to develop a trusting relationship with a provider, especially if you have not had a good experience within the healthcare system.** I have patients who experienced trauma in the form of sexual abuse as children or in violent intimate relationships and I didn't learn about it until they felt they had recovered enough to tell me. When I've asked if they waited to discuss their trauma because I had previously made them feel uncomfortable, their response has always been that it was not about me but that they were not ready. I then thank them for trusting me to share their experiences. I have learned over the years that patients who have experienced trauma are unaware that it can affect their physical and mental health later in life. The thing to know about trauma is that it can be generational, passed down from a grandparent to your parents and then to you and it can wreak its ugly head when you least expect it.

Your surgical history

Surgical history includes any operations you've had at any point in your life. Anything that was cut off, removed, replaced, enhanced, or biopsied under anesthesia is part of your surgical history. Often this information is placed under medical history because technically some surgeries are medical procedures. Many providers are only concerned about major surgeries and any complications you may have had. But if you had a breast biopsy, for example, even if it was benign (non-cancerous), a LEEP or cone biopsy for an abnormal pap smear, or a colonoscopy where a polyp was removed, it should be documented somewhere in your chart.

Were your tonsils or appendix removed when you were a child? Were your fallopian tubes tied/removed during a cesarean section? Did you have a hysterectomy and, if so, were the uterus, cervix, and fallopian tubes all removed or just one of these organs? Have you had thyroid surgery? Have you had your gallbladder removed?

Why are these surgeries important when they happened in the past? Because it tells your provider that these parts of your body should no longer cause problems. For example, if you presented with right sided abdominal pain and have already had your gallbladder (cholecystectomy is the medical term) removed, by reviewing your medical history, your provider would know that your symptoms are unrelated to your gallbladder.

Your social history

Social history includes all lifestyle choices that may affect your health. This includes information about your living situation; your level of education; what you do for work; smoking, alcohol and drug use (legal and not); and eating, sleeping, and exercise routines. It also includes how much you move during the day, how you control stress, and how you engage with others. During annual preventative health visits, I ask patients to walk me through a typical day in their lives from the time they get up to when they go to bed: what they eat, drink, how many minutes they get up and move, how active they are at work, and how many hours they sleep. Knowing this information helps me to better understand their lives and also suggest ways they can make small changes to get big results in their health.

When it comes to work, there are several issues that can affect your health: exposure to environmental chemicals, long or irregular shifts, night shifts, and long commutes.

In terms of your social life, it helps to know what your social connections are like and what you do for fun/leisure. Loneliness and social isolation are current public health problems that can have a negative impact on your health and well-being. But they are often not addressed during a healthcare visit. I have patients who have large extended families and friends but feel alone because they do not have true friends and people they trust to share their deepest concerns and struggles.

Level of education is important because it can indicate how well you will understand the questions asked and explanations provided. I have many immigrant patients who did not finish primary school, or people who went to school but still have difficulty comprehending medical information. Health illiteracy—the inability to understand and use health information to make informed decisions—is very common, especially when providers use terms learned in textbooks that may sound like a foreign language to you. I always ask patients if they understand and invite them to ask me for clarification. I speak Spanish, but my fluency in Spanish is not the same as English. When I am speaking Spanish with a patient, if I do not understand, I will ask for clarification and assume nothing.

Substance use is a significant health issue since it's on the rise, whether due to easier availability or mental health issues, such as addiction or loneliness. If you have a problem with substance use, it may make you feel better in the short term, numbing your pain, sending you to a more comfortable or interesting place, and taking your troubles away for a brief period. But mind-altering substances are also highly addictive, and the more you use, the more you need to get the same effect. Substance use can affect your personal and professional relationships and how well you meet your basic needs. Here are some of the most common substances that have a negative effect on your health:

- **Alcohol** includes beer, wine, and spirits (whiskey, bourbon, gin, vodka, brandy, tequila, etc.) and is easily accessible and tolerated by society. But drinking any alcoholic beverage in excess can negatively impact your health, both physical and mentally, especially if it contributes to missed work or relationship issues. Excessive alcohol use can also cause health problems affecting your heart, liver, and stomach and increase your cancer risk.

- **Marijuana** is now legal in many states and, as of the writing of this book, is illegal on a federal level. Buying marijuana from a dispensary is more expensive but at least you know that it hasn't been tainted with synthetic drugs like fentanyl. Marijuana today contains higher levels of THC—the psychoactive portion of the marijuana that gives marijuana the desired effect—which can have a more negative effect on your health than it did in the 1960s, when it was popularized as a recreational drug.

- **Tobacco** is well known for its harmful effects. Not only the addictive nature of the nicotine in tobacco but also the other chemicals in cigarettes that are harmful when breathed into our bodies. Tobacco can affect your blood vessels, increasing risk for developing high blood pressure and cardiovascular disease, including heart attack and stroke. Tobacco causes your skin to age faster and increases your cancer risk. Vaping/ e-cigarettes have been marketed as an alternative to cigarettes, adding flavor and taking away the smell of burning tobacco. While the exposure to many of the chemicals in cigarettes is reduced, vaping products still contain nicotine, which is addictive.

- **Opioids** are substances that attach to the opioid receptors in the brain, easing pain and causing good feelings. But the body can develop tolerance, requiring more opioids to induce pain relief and happiness. Taking any opioid regularly can cause severe withdrawal symptoms when stopped, leading to a dangerous pattern of increasing use and dosage to reduce pain, increase happiness, and avoid withdrawal symptoms. Many opioids, such as Oxycontin, which has caused much devastation for the past few decades, Vicodin, and Percocet are prescribed by health care providers and dentists. Kratom—known as gas station heroin—is legal and easily available at gas stations, smoke shops, stores and online because it is marketed as a supplement and not regulated. But kratom attaches to the opioid receptors in our brains, causing the same response as with other opioids, and should be avoided. There are illegal opioids, the most common being heroin and fentanyl, that can be purchased on the street. You can also purchase prescribed opioids illegally. The quantity of opioids in fentanyl is high, higher than what is legally prescribed, increasing risk of dependence after a single dose and overdose. Whenever possible, minimize your exposure to opioids and ask your PCP for alternatives for pain relief.

- **Other illicit drugs** that are stimulants include cocaine, crack cocaine, methamphetamines (meth), and MDMA (ecstasy). Drugs that cause hallucinations include PCP, psilocybin (mushrooms), LSD (acid), and ketamine. There is also an increase in the use of veterinarian tranquilizers mixed with opioids.

For your own health and safety, you need to be aware of what substances are out there, what risks they create, and how to safely avoid them or get off them if you've developed an addiction. If you have a history of substance use disorder, a mental health condition ranging from mild to severe (addiction), you may not be comfortable disclosing substance use to your PCP. I get it. You may be afraid your provider will judge you, and you may fear the consequences if you reveal what and how much you use. But substance use disorder is treatable. You should discuss your use with a professional to learn all your options. And it's important for you to understand that your PCP is dedicated to keeping your health information private. It may take several visits to develop trust with a provider before you are comfortable disclosing parts of yourself you may not feel like sharing. I hope for the sake of your health that it happens. Knowing this information makes it easier for your provider to create a plan for you to get to a better state of health and wellness.

If you or someone you know is struggling with substance use disorder, I have included resources at the end of the book for where to go for help.

The social side of health

Still not convinced that your social history is relevant to your health? Here is an example: You have uncontrolled blood pressure and were previously prescribed medication that contains hydrochlorothiazide (HCTZ), a medicine that makes you need to urinate. You were told to take it in the morning, but you do not take it because you work the night shift, and taking the medication in the morning keeps you from getting sleep because you are waking to use the toilet. Since you work the night shift, you often grab a deli sandwich and a bag of chips on your way to work to eat during your break.

Knowing you work the nightshift and that you generally eat salty chips and a sandwich with lunch meat that is high in salt, your provider would have a better understanding of why your blood pressure is not controlled. You may not need a higher dose of your blood pressure medication. Instead, you may need instruction on taking your medication at a different time of day and finding meal alternatives that are lower in salt. You may find that your blood pressure is well controlled just by tweaking these two things.

Your family history

It is important, to know your parents, siblings and grandparents' medical history. Why is this important? Your family history is like a crystal ball into your future life, and knowing it provides your PCP with the opportunity to educate you about potential health risks and what can be done to reduce your risk. If you have a genetic predisposition for certain illnesses (something hereditary), you can reduce but not eliminate your risk.

Here is the thing. Many providers do not obtain a full family health history and check the box for mother and father without completing this history. You then miss opportunities for education and screening. Knowing your history, your PCP can talk to you about your risks and when you need to begin screening for these potential issues. If your PCP, especially someone who you have never seen before, does not get a full family history, they put you at higher risk of not getting the screening tests you need when you need them. Screening finds illnesses early. Screening saves lives.

Examples of hereditary illnesses include:

- **High blood pressure:** If your parents and grandparents had high blood pressure and a brother has high blood pressure, chances are good that you have inherited the risk for high blood pressure. The same holds true for certain cancers: breast, ovarian, and colon. If you have a family history of one or the other, especially in a parent or sibling, your risk is higher.

- **Diabetes**: Sometimes referred to as sugar, diabetes is not necessarily hereditary, but if there is a strong family history (mother, father, grandparents, siblings), chances are that poor eating patterns were learned across generations—your mother learned to cook from your grandmother, and your mother taught you. If you grew up in a house where you ate a diet high in carbohydrates (think bread, rice, sweet bread, pancakes, tortillas, macaroni, noodles or other type of pasta and junk food) with few vegetables, chances are you still eat the same foods and have a higher risk of developing diabetes. But if you don't eat those foods, or eat smaller portions, and you are active, your chance of developing diabetes decreases. Just because your family has diabetes, does not mean you will develop it. You just have a higher risk than someone who doesn't have that history.

- **Addiction and mental health issues:** If your provider is concerned about something, knowing there is a family history of mental health issues can help them make a better diagnosis and treatment plan for you.

It is very important to know your own family history and share anything concerning with your PCP. However, if you do not know your parents or grandparents, because they died when you were young, you were adopted, or you do not communicate with them, that is okay. Knowing there are blanks in your family history helps us keep you on track for regular screenings when we don't know your health risks.

Patient Story

I met Talisha when she was 34. She was receiving treatment for breast cancer and had recurrent vaginal issues related to her treatment and the stress she was under because of it. She was a single mother of two girls. Her mother was also going through chemotherapy for breast cancer, but she did not test positive for either the BRCA 1 or BRCA 2 gene. A year after meeting Talisha, she referred her teenage daughter Quanella to me for birth control. Quanella had been seen at the clinic many times but nowhere in her chart was it recorded that there was a family history of breast cancer in her mother and maternal grandmother. As a teenager, it is rare that Quanella would develop breast cancer, but she is at high risk of developing breast cancer in her lifetime and I made sure this was documented in her family history and on the problem list on her chart for future reference. The electronic health record is permanent, it cannot get lost like a paper chart.

Your obstetric history

For women, your history of past pregnancies is important, especially if you had complications like blood pressure issues (gestational hypertension, preeclampsia, eclampsia), gestational diabetes, or cardiomyopathy. Complications in pregnancy can affect your future health risks and it is important to have it on record and be closely monitored as you age. But the pregnancy history is also important during your childbearing years—especially if you want to know if it is still possible to get pregnant again. If you are still getting a period and did not have any surgeries to prevent pregnancy, have not hit menopause, and are not using anything to prevent pregnancy,

pregnancy is still possible. Past pregnancy outcomes can affect a new pregnancy. You may have had an abortion or several abortions in the past and not be comfortable sharing that information with your provider or have it in the health record. That is ok, just keep that history tucked into your brain if it is ever needed.

Your menstrual history

For women, your menstrual history is important, especially if there has been a sudden change. The first day of your last period, your menstrual cycle, is a vital sign about your health status. Age at first period (menarche) can be a risk factor for health issues later in life if your first period was very early (8 or 9 years of age) or late (16 years of age or later). Early onset of menopause (when you are under age 40 and have not had a period in more than a year) and irregular periods (less or more than once a month) can also be risk factors. If your periods stop suddenly and you are a teenager or young woman in your 20s or early 30s, this is very concerning and warrants a discussion with your healthcare provider.

Sexual orientation and gender identity

Health Resources & Services Administration (HRSA) requires your PCP to ask about your sexual orientation and gender identity. The Centers for Medicare & Medicaid Services requires this information be placed in your EMR and updated, if needed. Why? Because your care should be centered around you. In a healthcare provider's office, you have the right to feel comfortable when you are most vulnerable, sharing personal aspects of your history and life, especially if your exam requires you to get undressed. Knowing who you are and how you identify is critical to providing you the best care.

Sexual history

Many patients and providers feel uncomfortable discussing sex, even though it is a natural human behavior. This discomfort is often due to societal taboos surrounding the topic, which can affect your sex life. Your sexual history includes the age at which you first started having sex, the number of lifetime partners you have had, your current number of partners, and what you are doing to prevent sexually transmitted infections if you are not in a monogamous relationship or are engaging in casual sex. Your provider can discuss ways to reduce the risk of sexually transmitted infections, such as PrEP, doxycycline, and condoms.

Are you planning or avoiding pregnancy and what methods are you using? If you do not plan to become pregnant soon and are not using a birth control method, your provider can discuss your options. Your sexual practices and reasons for not having sex, if applicable, are also important to discuss. If you are experiencing discomfort or pain during sex, it's important to talk to your provider, who can discuss options to help. Knowing that your sexual history is part of your health history may make it easier to talk about concerns. Also, know that if you are uncomfortable talking about your sexual history when your provider asks, just tell them that you don't want to talk about it.

Chapter Eleven

Your Vital Signs: Objective Information

After your PCP has reviewed your health history, the next part of the visit is the physical exam, which includes your vital signs and physical exam findings. This exam will depend on whether you are having your annual wellness visit or an illness visit. If you are having an annual wellness visit, you would have a more thorough exam. If you are seeing your women's health care provider, they are also able to do a complete exam, saving you an extra appointment with your PCP. If you are seeing the PCP for an illness or injury, the exam should focus on the problem you are presenting with.

This chapter covers all the objective information your PCP may assess during your visits.

Physical exam findings

The following parts of your body are frequently checked during an annual exam or when they are involved with your current health issue.

- **Head:** Your PCP will examine your ears, eyes, nose, throat, and thyroid gland.
- **Chest:** They will listen to your lungs and heart.
- **Abdomen:** They will examine the area below your ribs to above your pubic hair.
- **Reflexes:** They will test for normal reflexes by using a hammer or side of hand to gently tap your knee and/or your elbows or ankles.
- **Skin:** They will do a visual check for moles, rashes, skin discoloration, lesions

- **Cranial nerves:** They will examine your nervous system would include checking your cranial nerves.
- **Breasts:** If you are not having any breast complaints (mass, lump, skin discoloration, changes in the skin, nipple pain or discharge), your provider should ask you if you want a clinical breast exam. Your body, your choice.
- **Pelvic:** If you present with pelvic concerns such as vaginal discharge, odor, itching, feeling a sore or something unusual, or having pelvic pain, your provider will do a pelvic exam. Depending on your symptoms, this may involve a bi-manual exam (where they gently insert two lubricated gloved fingers in your vagina and examine your uterus and adnexa on either side (adnexa is the fallopian tube and ovaries), with another hand examining your lower abdomen right above your pubic hair line.
- **Prostate:** If you are a man over 50, your PCP may recommend a digital rectal exam where they gently insert a lubricated gloved finger into the rectum to feel the prostate gland for lumps.

Height and weight

Height and weight are used to calculate BMI (body mass index). This is not the best or most accurate measurement, but it provides a starting point to discuss health status, wellness, and health risks. BMI gives you a ballpark idea of where your weight should be in relation to your height but does not account for muscle mass. (It is more useful for healthcare providers to look at the ratio of your hip and waist measurements, but this is more difficult to calculate during your visit or by yourself.)

The Centers for Medicare & Medicaid Services (CMS) requires that your BMI is recorded in your health chart. I have attached a link to the National Institutes of Health's online BMI calculator in the Resources section of this book. A normal BMI is 18.5 to 24.9. Below 18.5 is underweight, 25 to 29.9 is considered overweight, and over 30 is classified as obese. (If you are a body builder with a BMI of 30 or over, eating healthy meals, and exercising and have little body fat, you may not have a medical issue. Muscle weighs more than fat. I would still recommend blood work to make sure all levels are normal.)

Weight can be a sensitive topic for many people and providers should handle it respectfully. While providers and patients alike are uncomfortable speaking about excess weight, obesity is a medical condition. Addressing weight is important for health and wellness. Remember, your healthcare provider's responsibility is to educate you about your health.

We all have fat tissue (the medical term is adipose tissue). Fat is the hormone highway system and we need it for our body to communicate with itself. Fat insulates our bodies and serves as a layer of protection for our internal organs and stores important vitamins. **Having too little or too much fat can cause illness.** Weight loss surgeries and medications have been developed to help treat obesity. **If you do not have a problem with obesity, you should not be prescribed these treatments.**

More times than not, obesity is caused by high intake of fast, convenient, and processed foods combined with inactivity. Your PCP may have a conversation with you about your lifestyle and eating habits to help you understand your health risks and how you can work towards a better state of health and wellness. Blood work should be done to screen for metabolic disorders (these include diabetes and heart disease).

If your BMI is over 30, your PCP should ask you the following questions: Are you preparing your meals at home from scratch? Are you eating three to four servings of vegetables each day? Are you eating fruits, seeds and nuts, lean protein like fish, chicken, and eggs? How about beans or lentils? Are you avoiding processed, pre-made and junk foods, limiting your alcohol intake, and not smoking? Is your intake of sweetened beverages like juices and pop/soda low? Are you engaging in aerobic exercise and strength training and avoiding sitting for most of your waking hours? Do you sleep at least 7 hours each night?

If, during your typical day, you eat most of your meals outside of the home or heat up meals you bought in a box or from the freezer section of the grocery store and your BMI is 30 or higher, your PCP can recommend modifications and may also refer you to a dietician for further support.

Obesity increases the risk of developing diabetes, heart disease, joint pain, and possibly cancer to name a few illnesses. This is not just Bad News Barbara trying to scare you. Research proves this to be true. Read more about how you can lower your health risks in Chapter Sixteen: Eat. Move. Rest. Repeat. You will be amazed at how easy and affordable it can be to live a healthy lifestyle.

Blood pressure

Blood pressure is the amount of force needed to pump blood throughout your body. Your blood pressure should ideally remain below 120/80. The top reading, systolic blood pressure, is a measure of the pressure your body uses when the heart beats. The bottom reading, diastolic blood pressure, is a measurement of pressure when your body is at rest. Hypertension, commonly called high blood pressure, is a silent killer around the world. Many people do not know they have high blood pressure and often there are no symptoms. **Uncontrolled high blood pressure can lead to a heart attack, stroke, kidney disease and more.**

Unfortunately, I am seeing younger people with high blood pressures in the 130s/80s or 140s/90s refusing interventions. As a PCP, I can educate and point out the health issues, but I have to let my patients make their own decisions about their health.

The Silent Threat: A Patient's Battle with Uncontrolled Hypertension

I have many patients like Allison. She is 29 and her blood pressure is consistently 150s/100s at her visits. She makes appointments with me but insists she has no complaints and reports she feels fine. She has a family history of hypertension, with her mother, father, two sisters, and both maternal and paternal grandparents having suffered from it. Her mother had her first stroke at age 45 and died from a heart attack at age 55. Her father died from a heart attack at age 56. Allison's body mass index is 50 (this is class 3 obesity).

Allison does not cook, eats mostly fast food, is not active during the day. She sleeps nine to ten hours each night. She refuses medication. I have offered a referral to bariatric surgery, not specifically to have the surgery but to get the nutritional and emotional support I think she needs to make lifestyle changes. I worry that she will have a heart attack or stroke, develop kidney failure, need dialysis or worse, die an early death.

There have been visits when I bring up my concern about her blood pressure and she tells me, "I made an appointment for another reason, I did not come here to talk about my blood pressure." Noted. I express my concerns, write in her chart that she is aware of her risks, and that she is not receptive to counseling and declines treatment. I cannot make her do anything. I can continue to offer counseling and be there when she is ready. Her body. Her choice. Her health. There must be a reason why she continues to make appointments with me. I hope she knows my fussing is because I care.

I care especially because high blood pressure is personal to me. I live a healthy lifestyle, am a vegetarian, could be less high strung but working on it by meditating multiple times per day and exercising, and my blood work is normal. But I have a family history of heart disease, hypertension, and stroke. To reduce my risk of developing a stroke, having a heart attack, or other consequences of uncontrolled high blood pressure, I know I need to take medication, but also to continue with my healthy lifestyle and do better at controlling my stress. My PCP discussed the side effects of medications with me. One had a possible side effect of cough, and because I have asthma, work in healthcare and am exposed to respiratory infections, I opted for a different medication. It took several visits before my blood pressure was controlled, but the plan was created by my PCP and me. Shared decision-making. Though I understand high blood pressure as a clinician, I went to the Mayo Clinic's website to understand it as a patient.

Pulse and respirations

Pulse is the number of times your heart beats in one minute. The average pulse rate is 60 to 100 beats per minute and is a measurement of heart health. We check pulse to make sure your heart isn't working too much or not well enough. Pulse gives us information about your fitness level, blood circulation, heart rhythm, thyroid health, and overall heart health.

Respirations are the number of breaths you take in one minute. The normal range is 12 to 16 breaths per minute. We assess whether you are breathing too fast or your breathing is low and labored. Abnormal breathing patterns can signal respiratory diseases or disorders, including neurological issues.

Temperature

Your body temperature is a vital sign that can quickly indicate the presence of infection or inflammation in the body. An elevated temperature— fever—can be a sign of various conditions ranging from minor viral infections to more serious illnesses, while an abnormally low temperature might suggest hypothermia or other health issues. The average human body temperature is 98.6 degrees F (37 C). A fever is over 99 F (37.2 C).

Last menstrual period

The first day of your last menstrual period (not the last day) is an important vital sign that is often overlooked in primary care. Irregular periods can be a cause for concern, not only in terms of fertility and pregnancy but other health issues. Once you stop having periods, either because you are post-menopause or for some other reason, some health risks, especially for heart disease and osteoporosis increase.

Pain levels

Pain is a driving force for substance use disorder, both opioid and alcohol use. Too often, pain is not properly addressed during PCP visits—for many people, but especially people of color. Pain can be physical or emotional, but both are equally relevant and affect your health. Life is hard and some people find numbing the pain is easier to get through life than facing the pain head on.

By understanding the components of your physical exam, you can be a more active participant in your healthcare, engaging more effectively with your healthcare provider. Remember, the physical exam is not just a routine procedure, but a crucial tool in maintaining your health and catching potential issues early.

Chapter Twelve

———

Objective Assessments: Tests and Screenings

Laboratory tests and screenings are vital tools in modern healthcare, providing crucial information about your body's internal functions and potential health risks. These tests can range from routine blood work to ultrasound exams to computed tomography (CT) scans, each offering unique insights into your health status. Understanding what these tests are looking for and why they're ordered is essential for active participation in your healthcare journey. This knowledge not only helps you make informed decisions but also enables you to ask relevant questions and better interpret your results.

In this chapter, we'll explore common lab tests and screenings, their purposes, and what their results might mean for your overall health.

Typical lab tests

If your PCP orders **lab tests or blood work**, ask to have the tests explained and why you need them. Your PCP has to relate any tests they order with a diagnosis for insurance to cover the cost of it. Many tests are ordered as a preventative measure, to screen for a potential health disorder early, such as high cholesterol, colorectal cancer, prostate cancer, or pre-diabetes. Others are meant to confirm a diagnosis, such anemia, diabetes, a yeast infection, a *sexually transmitted infection, or cancer.*

You should be agreeing to all tests that are ordered. For example, when I have a patient with diabetes who is due for their hemoglobin A1C (HgbA1c) test, an average measurement of blood sugar, I will offer the test. That way, when she next sees her diabetes specialist (known as an endocrinologist), they will already have current information. I have had patients who decline the test, not wanting to know their current levels because they know they haven't been doing a good job of managing their condition. As important as the test is, it is their body. Their choice. Their health. I document that I offered the test and they declined. I must respect their decision not to want the test.

If you want to be tested for something the provider has not mentioned, don't hesitate to ask if the test can be done and if it should be covered by insurance. For example, given that I work in women's health, many people come requesting a STI (sexually transmitted infection) screening. I never order an STI screening for everyone, making the assumption they need it. But I generally ask about the person's sexual activity, because it can affect their health. STI's like chlamydia can cause problems later in life (increase cervical cancer risk, infertility). Not all PCPs will bring up the subject. But if you are having sex without a condom with a new partner and don't know their STI status or with a partner you do not trust, or if you have multiple sex partners, you are at risk for STIs and should ask to get screened. If you are in a committed relationship, have never had an STI, and your risk is low for STIs, you do not necessarily need screening unless you want it.

You can also decline screening. Just because a test is available does not necessarily mean that it needs to be ordered. Before you agree to any tests, you should have a conversation about what tests are being offered, what the PCP will you do with the information, how it might change your care plan, and how much you will need to pay for the test if it is not covered by your insurance.

It is common for a PCP to order the following blood tests at your annual preventive health visit. If you are given access to your lab (blood work) results, those results will include the normal range as a reference point. If your results fall above or below what is considered normal, it should be highlighted or in bold type face. Your PCP will take your results into context, based on whether the test is preventive (to detect an issue before you show symptoms), meant to detect the cause of your presenting complaint, or used to manage a chronic health condition.

CBC—The Complete Blood Count checks your red and white blood cells to check for infection or anemia (low red blood cells). There are many parts to the CBC, with multiple indicators measuring red and white blood cells.

CMP—The Comprehensive Metabolic Panel checks sugar, protein, kidney, and liver functions. Some PCPs will only order a BMP (basic metabolic panel) that does not check liver function. Many illnesses (heart disease, kidney disease, non-alcoholic fatty liver, and diabetes) are metabolic in nature. That's a fancy term for things that naturally happen within your body based on the foods you eat. The incidence of nonalcoholic fatty liver (medically named steatotic liver disease) is relatively high. If you have risk factors, such as a family history of the disease, high cholesterol, metabolic syndrome, insulin resistance, or obesity, ask for the CMP if you see that only a BMP has been ordered.

HgBA1C (Hemoglobin A1C): This checks for diabetes (basically, your sugar level over the past 6 to 8 weeks). It is an important measurement to determine pre-diabetes or how well controlled your diabetes is if you have diabetes. Normal measurements are below 5.5. A measurement of 5.6 to 6.3 indicates pre-diabetes (meaning without lifestyle changes you will develop diabetes), and anything over 6.4 is diabetes. If you are a diabetic, the goal is to have an HgBA1C value below 7.0.

Lipid panel: The lipid panel has 4 major values, and your overall cardiovascular risk is determined by all values taken together:

- Total cholesterol
- HDL (High-Density Lipoprotein, the "good" cholesterol that protects the heart)
- Triglycerides (a type of fat in the blood)
- LDL (Low-Density Lipoprotein, often called "bad" cholesterol)

A normal total cholesterol level is below 200. There's often a relationship between high triglycerides and high HbA1c, which can be related to a diet high in carbohydrates (bread, cereal, pasta, tortillas, cookies, crackers, cookies, processed foods, and added sugars). While I have patients who are told they have high cholesterol when their totals are in the low 200s, it's important to look at the ratio between LDL and HDL. A normal HDL level is anything above 40. Even if the LDL is slightly elevated, a high HDL can offset this risk. The LDL/HDL ratio is calculated by dividing the LDL by the HDL. A ratio below 3.5 is generally considered good, with lower ratios indicating lower cardiovascular risk. Small tweaks to your diet can lower a slightly elevated LDL while maintaining the protective high HDL.

Thyroid studies (usually a TSH, T3, T4, sometimes reflex TPO antibodies): Thyroid disorders are very common in women. If your chief complaint suggests a thyroid issue, your provider will order this test. If you have a family history and are having symptoms related to thyroid disorders, this test will also be ordered.

HIV testing is recommended once in a lifetime, as is Hepatitis C screening—more often if you have risk factors.

Sexually Transmitted Infection (STI) screenings: If you are at risk (sexually active with multiple partners, new partner, do not trust your current partner or are just concerned), you should ask for this screening. Blood tests are used to screen for HIV, syphilis (RPR), and Hepatitis B. Samples for gonorrhea, chlamydia, and trichomoniasis can be taken from urine, mouth, vagina, and/or anus depending on sexual activity and exposure. Testing for herpes simplex (HSV) should only occur if you have an actual sore/lesion, since blood tests for HSV can be inaccurate.

Gynecology (well woman) exam tests

The above lab tests should be ordered during your annual wellness exam, but that depends on your provider. If you are having your annual gynecology exam, your women's healthcare provider may order a pap smear (a screening test for cervical cancer) or vaginal cultures to check for bacterial vaginosis, candida (yeast infection), and/or sexually transmitted infections.

To save yourself time, you can ask your women's health care provider to order the typical lab tests as well. If they don't provide primary care but can give you an order for the tests, your PCP can review your lab results when you see them next. You will have access through the patient portal to show your PCP the results if their electronic medical record does not integrate with the lab where the tests were done.

Chronic illness screenings

If you are managing a chronic condition like diabetes, hypertension, kidney disease, heart failure, or thyroid disease you may need a hemoglobinA1C every 3 months, especially if your diabetes/sugar is not well controlled. For diabetes and high blood pressure conditions, your provider may also order urine studies to check kidney function like the microalbumin/creatinine ratio. It never hurts to ask your provider what tests you are due for to make sure everything is functioning the way it should.

Specific tests for individual health problems

Your PCP may order specific tests to determine whether you are experiencing symptoms that might suggest a urinary tract infection (very common in women, rarer for men), or sexually transmitted infection testing (STI). Other tests can be performed to diagnose vaginal odor or irritation, low energy, or excessive tiredness. There are a lot of reasons for blood work.

One important test that is often overlooked is used to detect h. pylori, a bacteria found in the gut that can cause ulcers, gastritis (inflammation in the stomach) and, if left untreated, stomach cancer. **If you have signs of h. pylori infection such as stomach pain or burning, nausea, decreased appetite, or bloating, talk to your PCP about ordering this test.** Some of my patients who have tested positive for this condition report worsening pain in the lower abdomen after they eat or discomfort all over their abdomens. Typically, this is a 15-minute breath test, but sometimes your stool is tested. If your test is positive, you will receive two weeks of antibiotics (if you are prone to getting yeast infections with antibiotic use, and many women are, ask for yeast medication with refills). Trust me on this one. I tested positive for h. pylori about 20 years ago and had the worse yeast infection of my life! I would not wish that on anyone! I now give a prescription for terconazole-3 with 1 refill for anyone testing positive for h. pylori. Unlike other tests, if you test positive for h. pylori you need to be re-tested one to two months after you complete your antibiotics to make sure that the infection has been treated appropriately and to prevent complications.

Screening milestones

There are several screenings that you should consider having regularly. The most common are pap smears and mammograms for women, prostate screenings for men, and colonoscopies for both women and men. Since you may not see the same doctor from year to year, you should know why these screenings are important and how often you need them.

Pap smears (cervical smear)

A pap smear was originally designed to test for cervical cancer. Cervical cancer tends to be a slow growing cancer, but if caught early, it can be treated. Today pap smears may also be collected from the throat and anus to check for cancers caused by the same strains of the HPV virus (human papilloma virus). This virus is the most common sexually transmitted infection. If you have never had sex, your risk for developing cervical cancer is low.

As of the writing of this book, pap smears generally are first done at age 21 (the assumption is that all women have had sex by this time). If you have never had sex and are 21 or older, you may not need the test or can decline it knowing your risk is low. Generally, pap smears are not done after age 65, since the risk of HPV developing into cervical cancer is low. However, if you are 65 and haven't had a pap smear since you were 50, you might ask for one. Also, if you have a history of abnormal pap smears, pap smears should continue for 20 years after your last normal one, or until age 65. So, if you had an abnormal pap smear and your last normal one was at age 50, you need pap smears until age 70.

Since collecting the smear is invasive and can be uncomfortable—especially for women who have never had vaginal penetration—you should talk to your PCP or women's healthcare provider about whether you really need a pap smear. Express any concerns you have. The pap smear can also be uncomfortable and traumatic for someone who has experienced sexual trauma. Creating a calm and caring environment for this procedure is crucial for developing a patient's trust. Many women have had traumatic experiences having a pap smear and forego their care until they experience real problems. This is where shared decision making with your provider is important. It is ok to decline. Your body, your choice, your health. All providers can do is counsel and document. Your provider should document the conversation in your health record so the next time they (or someone else) see you, they know your concerns.

There is good information on the horizon. In May 2024, the FDA approved an HPV test that allows for self-collection in a healthcare setting for women 25 and older.[15] These tests are already in use in other countries, but new to the US, and will reduce the barriers that come with having a pap smear. The tests should be widely available in most outpatient care settings for insured and uninsured women in the Fall of 2024. If you are due for screening, ask your provider about the new tests. Many providers may be hesitant to use the new tests (as much as they were when we moved from conventional pap smears to the ThinPrep) but this is a gamechanger to get more women screened for cervical cancer. Timing of screenings will also change with this test to every 5 years between ages 25 and 65 with a negative HPV test.[16]

Mammograms

A mammogram is an x-ray exam of your breasts to screen for breast cancer. Mammogram screening saves lives. However, there is debate over when screening should begin and how often you should have one. Some organizations say you should have your first one at 40, others say 50. My professional opinion is age 40.

Your insurance will pay for a mammogram once you are 40 but you might want to discuss the need with your provider. They can counsel you on your risk of breast cancer based on family history and other factors. If you have a family history in a first degree relative (mom or sister), screening should start 10 years earlier than the age at your family member's breast cancer diagnosis. For example, if a mother or sister was 45 when they were diagnosed with breast cancer, your mammogram should start at age 35. Also, Black and Latina women tend to be diagnosed with breast cancer at an earlier age then white women and tend to have more aggressive types of breast cancer.[17] I started getting mammograms at age 27 because I felt a lump that concerned me and my mother died from breast cancer at the age of 30 (she was diagnosed when she was 28). In my case, screening should have begun at age 18, but most organizations will not do a mammogram that early.

If you are over 40, have never had a mammogram, and your provider does not bring it up, ask for it. Except for one patient who was in her mid 60s when I diagnosed her breast cancer, my other breast cancer patients have all been in their 40s. In some practices, the care gap notification for breast cancer screening appears at age 50. If this is the case, a provider may not order a mammogram if you are younger than 50. Most insurances will pay for a mammogram after 40 and you have the right to ask for it.

Now, with tomosynthesis mammography, which uses low-dose x-rays, mammograms are more comfortable than they used to be. It may take you five to six months before you can get a mammogram appointment, especially if you live in an under-resourced urban or rural community. Imagine being told by your PCP the importance of mammogram screening only to be told by the imaging center that you have to wait months to get one. Like I said earlier, there are many problems in healthcare today.

Colorectal cancer screening (aka colon cancer screening)

The colon and rectum are the last part of your digestive system where your food travels before you poop (what goes into your mouth will be peed out, sweated out, pooped out, or stored).

Colorectal cancer rates are increasing particularly in younger people. [18] Experts say it has to do with a number of factors, including high antibiotic use, which negatively affects the gut microbiome, diet, low natural fiber diets (not enough vegetables, fruits, whole grains, beans), processed foods, and inactivity.

This is where I become Bad News Barbara, because the future is scary when looking at health trends. What you eat today will affect you today, tomorrow and the rest of your life. I tell my patients that if you eat crap, you feel like crap, and you can't crap, which can increase your risk of illness, including colorectal cancer. If you are not having a bowel movement every day, look at what you are eating and make sure you include natural fiber in your diet.

The newest recommendation for when to have your first colorectal cancer screening has changed to age 45. If you have a family history of colorectal cancer or other risk factors, your PCP may recommend you have one earlier.

If you are younger than 45 and having symptoms that might indicate a problem, talk to your PCP. Constipation, diarrhea, blood in your stool or blood on the toilet paper after you wipe, chronic hemorrhoids, and persistent cramping in your lower abdomen can be related to a colorectal issue. There are simple lab tests that can be ordered (fecal occult or FIT test or Cologuard, depending on availability and whether it is covered by your insurance). But if there is cause for concern and/or family history, ask for a referral to a gastroenterologist (a specialist in the digestive tract) to discuss whether you need a colonoscopy. Though colonoscopies are invasive, if something unusual (a polyp) is seen, it can be removed, reducing your cancer risk.

Prostate screening

This blood test for men checks for something called prostate specific antigen (PSA), which can be high if you have prostate problems. An elevated PSA can indicate a problem ranging from benign prostatic hyperplasia (BPH), which is the noncancerous swelling of the prostate, to prostate cancer. There is controversy in the medical field about whether this test is necessary, so it's important to talk to your provider about it first. A family history of prostate cancer or an inconclusive digital rectal exam may justify having the test. Some people say it can lead to extra tests, costs, and worry for no reason.

Lung cancer screening

If you are a smoker or have a history of long-term cigarette smoking, talk with your provider about having a chest x-ray to screen for lung cancer.

Osteoporosis screening

If you are 65 or older (female or male) or have other risks factors for fractures, talk to your provider about your fracture risk and ordering a bone density test.

Chapter Thirteen

―――

Your Body Talks to You: Why You Should Listen.

Believe in the power of the human body—of your body. Your body talks to you. Not the way some people with psychiatric illness hear voices. But in general, your body talks to you by having physical symptoms.

Understanding and interpreting your own body's signals is key to managing your health. Listen to your body. Tune into your symptoms, ask yourself questions, write down your answers, and see if they give you any insights as to why you have this problem. If you can't solve the situation on your own, take your answers with you when you see your provider for a professional diagnosis and treatment plan. I recommend you resist the urge to search your complaints online. You can always find a list of medical conditions associated with your symptoms, but you will lose your mind body connection. You may also learn information that is irrelevant to your situation.

On a side note, there is a lot of useful information online and I do encourage my patients to go to the Mayo Clinic, Cleveland Clinic, or CDC websites to validate the information that we've discussed during their visit if they want more information. Sometimes people learn better when they can read or watch videos or see graphics rather than listening. (I will provide links to their pages in the resources section at the end of the book.) These websites will often show up at the top of your search results.

Of course, you can do your own search online for the conditions that might ail you, and you may find information that contradicts the reputable healthcare sites. That may feel good if the information on those reputable sites is negative. It's human nature to shy away from bad news and believe if you don't think about it, the problem will go away. However, when it comes to our health, knowing the bad stuff can be motivating to change behaviors and make healthcare appointments. When it comes to healthcare, the things to be concerned about often do not go away and if left untreated can progress to something worse.

Below is a list of the most common complaints patients have and the questions you can ask yourself if you are experiencing any of them. This list is not exhaustive, but reading these examples should give you a better understanding of how to listen to your body and the questions to ask yourself and answer. Chances are, if you experience any of these issues, you'll have to wait for your next provider appointment, unless you go to immediate or urgent care. In the meantime, you can problem solve on your own and if your symptoms remain unchanged, your provider may be able to use the answers to these questions to diagnose the cause of your complaint.

Please refer to the list in Chapter Seven for symptoms that require emergency care—and don't ignore those!

Headaches

Many patients present with complaints of frequent headaches. You may suffer from migraines. The headache may be related to sinuses. But look at your headaches from a different perspective and consider other causes. When was the last time you had your eyes checked? Were you prescribed glasses/contact lenses but do not wear them? How much time do you spend in front of a screen (computer, phone, tablet, television)? How many hours are you sleeping each night? What is your stress level? What are you eating? Are you eating enough? What is your water intake and is it possible you are dehydrated? When in the day do they occur? Are you sensitive to sound or light? Do you have other symptoms around your headaches like nausea or visual disturbances? What makes them better? Or worse?

Back pain

If you are having pain along your spine in the area between your neck and shoulders, this may be related to stress or to the amount of time you spend hunched over your phone or computer. Lower back pain is the more common back pain. Have you started a new exercise routine? When you bend down to pick up something or lift something heavy, are you lifting with your back or with your legs? Weak thigh, buttocks, and abdominal muscles and incorrect body mechanics can lead to lower back pain. I tell my patients if we were meant to lift things with our back, we would have four legs. Bad posture can also cause low back pain. So can the number of pillows you sleep with at night. How old is your mattress? Do you toss and turn at night? These things can also cause lower back pain. We should be spending 30% of our lives sleeping but if we are twisting our spines at night, we may be contributing to back pain. What have you taken or done to ease the pain? Does stretching help or make it worse? Does the pain radiate upwards or downwards?

Chest Pain

Do you have a racing heartbeat that comes and goes? You may have gone to the emergency room or had many tests only to be told that everything is normal. But you do not feel normal. Are you feeling anxiety and stress? Panic attacks are common and can present themselves in many ways, chest pain being a common complaint when someone is having a panic attack. (I have included signs and symptoms of a heart attack and stroke in the resources section.)

Shortness of breath

Are you short of breath and have other symptoms? Are you short of breath when you climb a flight or two of stairs? When you exercise? When wheezing? Does the shortness of breath occur when you are feeling nervous? Does taking three to five deep breaths make it go away? Is it worse when you are outside—do you live near a freeway, factory, or garbage dump—places that contribute to air pollution?

Abdominal pain

Abdominal pain can be a symptom of various conditions, ranging from minor to life-threatening. Does your pain come and go? Is it related to anything you ate? Have you been drinking water regularly so you're well hydrated? Does the pain only occur after you eat? Does it occur when you are stressed? Some people have a gut punch reaction to stress. Do any over-the-counter medications help? What, if anything, makes it better? Are you experiencing other symptoms like nausea, vomiting, diarrhea or constipation? Do you have a fever? Chills? In some cases, abdominal pain may require a visit to the emergency department. Call your provider's office and speak with an advice nurse or healthcare provider if your symptoms worsen. Keep a food diary until your appointment. When you see your provider ask if it's appropriate to have an h. pylori breath test. Often there is a relationship between what you eat and how you feel. People develop food sensitives or intolerance, especially to dairy and wheat products, as they age.

Lower abdominal pain and pelvic pain:

If you have a uterus and ovaries, does the pain happen two weeks after the first day of your last menstrual period? Could it be ovulation pain? Does it occur when you are stressed? Often people have a gut reaction to stress. How often do you poop? If you poop infrequently, do you feel better after you poop? Does the pain come and go? Do you have diarrhea? Gas? Do certain foods like dairy products make it worse? Is it persistent, do you have a new sexual partner? Do you have fever or chills?

Knee pain

This is a common ailment as you age and the cartilage in your knee joint breaks down—like wear and tear. But knee pain is often caused by inflammation as well. How active are you? Did you twist your knee recently? Did you play a lot of sports when you were younger? What makes it worse? What makes it better? If you are carrying extra weight around your midsection and are on your feet a lot, your knees are supporting that weight and could be causing your pain. What are you eating? Is your diet high in processed foods? These could be causing inflammation and make the pain worse.

Urinary tract infection (UTI)—aka bladder infection

Are you using the toilet more frequently? Do you feel like you need to go, but when you get to the toilet, nothing comes out? Does it hurt when you pee? Does it feel like you have emptied your bladder but then feel discomfort? Or feel like there is more urine to let out but then nothing comes out? Have you increased your water intake? Are you drinking energy drinks? Caffeinated drinks? Have you increased your intake of alcohol? The bladder has muscle memory and if you're filling it more than you had in the past, you may be using the toilet more. Many drinks can irritate the bladder and cause you to go more often? Do you hold your urine when you need to go? Are you not drinking enough? If you have a vagina, have you had sex with a new partner? Do you use the toilet after sex? Do you have anal sex and then vaginal sex? Do you wipe from front to back after using the toilet? This can often cause UTIs as the urethra (where you pee from), the vagina (where you have sex), and the anus (where you poop), are all close together and there are bacteria living in each system.

124

Vaginal itching

In people with vaginas, sometimes UTIs mimic vaginal itching (because the urethra/pee hole) is close to the vagina and more people experience yeast infections than UTIs. Are you having a change in vaginal discharge? Is it clumpy? Yellow-green in color? Change in odor (we all smell down there but does it smell like yeast—like if you were making bread?) (for all you bread bakers out there, I probably ruined the experience for you). Is it hot where you live and you sweat? Do you wear cotton crotched panties? Tight pants? Wear panty liners all day? Use a new soap, detergent?

Fatigue/lack of energy

What is your stress level? What are you eating? Are you eating enough? How many hours are you sleeping? Are you feeling sad, hopeless, depressed or lonely? Are you feeling fatigued at the same time every day? What did you eat hours before? As I said before and will say again, there is a relationship between what we eat and how we feel. If you are tired a couple of hours after lunch, then you may not have eaten a nutrient dense meal. I will say more on this in Chapter Sixteen, Eat. Move. Rest. Repeat.

Skin conditions

Blotchy skin, acne, skin discoloration, rashes, itching— most of these conditions are caused by inflammation. Think about the foods you are eating. Many cause inflammation, including on your skin. Are your food choices highly processed? Greasy? Have you used a new soap or body lotion? Makeup? New detergent or fabric softener? Bought a new piece of clothing without washing it first?

If you go through your list of questions for each complaint and can answer yes to any of them, you may have found the cause of your problem. Try eliminating that behavior and see if the problem doesn't solve itself on its own. If the problem doesn't go away and/or gets worse, don't hesitate to call your PCP's advice nurse and make an appointment if necessary. If they can't see you and you don't have an issue that requires emergency care, take yourself to urgent care.

Chapter Fourteen

Common Medical Conditions That Can Shorten Your Lifespan

Chronic health conditions or diseases lead to decreased life expectancy, and to a ball and chain relationship with medications. You are only given one life to live and it is up to you to make the decision to live life to its fullest.

Remember, everything you do today affects you today, tomorrow and the rest of your life. If you make bad choices concerning your health now, it can have devastating effects for your future. While living in the present is important for mental well-being, it's crucial to consider how your current lifestyle affects your long-term health. Neglecting healthy habits can lead to a cascade of health issues:

1. Your body may become resistant to medications, requiring higher doses or additional prescriptions.
2. Chronic illnesses can develop, potentially causing irreversible damage to organ systems.
3. These issues often compound, creating a snowball effect of declining health.

Lifestyle encompasses various factors that influence your well-being, including diet, physical activity, sleep patterns, and stress management. By making conscious, healthy choices in these areas, you can significantly reduce your risk of developing common chronic diseases. The following list, while not exhaustive, covers the most prevalent health conditions that people often face due to lifestyle factors.

Pre-diabetes and Diabetes (aka sugar)

Prediabetes is when your body is at risk of developing diabetes, but the disease is still preventable. There are two types of diabetes, Type 1 and Type 2. Type 1 is rarer and is an autoimmune disorder. (An autoimmune disorder is when your body's defense system, which usually fights off germs, gets confused and attacks your own healthy cells instead. It's like your body's army mistakenly seeing some of your own cells as invaders and trying to get rid of them.)

Type 2 diabetes is often caused by diet and lifestyle choices, which means it can be prevented. In this type of diabetes your body has trouble breaking down sugar from the foods you eat. Why is this important? Your body breaks down the food you eat into sugar (glucose) for energy.

Your pancreas makes a hormone called insulin, which helps your cells use this sugar. In Type 2 diabetes, your body either doesn't make enough insulin or doesn't use it well. This causes sugar to build up in your blood instead of being used by your cells. Diabetes can affect many different systems in your body, including your eyes, heart, kidneys, and toes.

Type 2 diabetes is caused by eating too many carbohydrates over time (think sweet foods like ice cream and soda but also starchy foods, like bread, pasta, and cereals). Even if these foods don't taste sweet, your body breaks them down into sugar. Eating too many carbs over time can overwhelm your body's ability to process sugar.

Type 2 diabetes is completely preventable. Of course you can treat diabetes with medication, but over time, if you do not control the amount of sugar you eat and how much you move throughout the day, your medications will stop working. At that point, you will need dialysis—when you need a machine to rid your body of waste and fluid (basically the machine functions as your kidneys). If you've been told you have prediabetes or worry that you are not controlling your diabetes well enough, I have included more diabetes information in the resources section.

Hypertension

Hypertension is commonly known as high blood pressure. It is a condition that occurs when the arteries or blood vessels create pressure, forcing the heart to work harder to pump blood throughout your body.

You may be staying to yourself, "I can just take medication to control that." But the human body is smarter than we are. If lifestyle changes are not made, the body becomes resistant. Your risk for a heart attack and stroke increases. Unmanaged high blood pressure can cause kidney damage, increasing your chance of needing dialysis. When this occurs, the damage is irreversible—you will need to rely on dialysis until you can get a kidney transplant.

Your provider should talk to you about your hypertension risk. This is another reason why it is important to know your family history. High blood pressure is often caused by lifestyle factors: smoking, not being active, and eating a diet high in fast and prepared foods and low in vegetables and other plants. But hypertension can also be hereditary—if you have a strong family history, chances are you may develop high blood pressure.

Remember I spoke about reducing risk? You can reduce your risk for hypertension but not eliminate it. If you have high blood pressure and you are doing everything right, taking your prescribed medication everyday along with maintaining a healthy lifestyle will reduce your risk of stroke and heart attack.

Heart Disease

Also known as cardiovascular disease, heart disease is the number one cause of death for women. Ironic isn't? We have big compassionate hearts and for many of us, our hearts are what fail us in the end. The best way to avoid heart disease is to ensure a healthy lifestyle. Eat a healthy diet, limiting processed foods. Exercise regularly. Maintain a healthy weight so you don't put a strain on your heart muscle. Don't smoke. Drink alcohol only in moderation. Manage your stress and get enough sleep.

If you have a chronic health condition, work with your provider to keep it under control. And if you have a family history of heart disease, get regular checkups. Small changes can make a big difference in your heart health over time. It's never too early or too late to start taking care of your heart!

Cancer

Cancers can develop in any part of the body and happen when normal cells develop into abnormal cells. According to the American Cancer Society, breast, prostate, endometrial (uterine), pancreatic, kidney, and melanoma (skin) cancers are on the rise and cancer is affecting younger generations.[19] Lifestyle and obesity are major contributing factors. In fact, in a recent study, 17 of the 24 most common cancers are increasing in young adults aged 25 to 49 and 10 of 17 cancers are related to obesity.[20] While environmental exposures like pollution and forever chemicals contribute to the problem, you can lower your own risk through weight management.

When it comes to skin cancers like melanoma, people underestimate their risk. Everyone who is exposed to the sun is at risk for skin cancer, regardless of skin color. Wearing sun block, covering your head with a hat, and minimizing your sun exposure (especially in the middle of the day when your exposure to UV rays is high) will reduce your cancer risk and keep you looking younger! Sun is a great way to get vitamin D, but my advice is to limit this exposure to 15 minutes max without sunblock. Any more time will increase your risk of sun burn, particularly if you have lighter skin.

Anxiety and depression

Anxiety and depression are rising, in younger generations but also in every generation. Mental health issues were made worse during the COVID pandemic because people were isolated from family, friends, and co-workers.

We are social by nature and meant to be connected by communities. But the world is changing. Family dynamics change as people move away for school or work, leaving their family and friends behind. It can be difficult to develop new relationships, especially as adults.

You may be engaging on social media and have many followers and connections but feel these relationships are not deep and meaningful, leaving you feeling socially isolated and lonely. We are so connected to our phones that we are forgetting to connect personally with one another. Loneliness is a public health crisis that many providers overlook. It can negatively impact your health.

Recognizing the importance of genuine human connection and actively building a supportive community are crucial steps in combating the rising tide of anxiety, depression, and loneliness, ultimately contributing to better overall health and well-being. It may take a village to raise a child, but it also takes the same village to support each other throughout our lives. If you are dealing with anxiety or depression, read the next chapter for more information on mental health and how to optimize it.

Chapter Fifteen

———

Mental Health is as Important as Physical Health

The terms mental health and behavioral health are used interchangeably. Mental health is anything that affects your mood and your physical and mental well-being. Childhood trauma, stress, anxiety, depression, loneliness, grief, and life in general can interfere with your mental health.

Life is hard and it gets harder the older we get because we have more responsibilities. Relationships are more complicated than they were in childhood. You may be uncomfortable talking about mental health because it was never talked about in your family while you were growing up (or even now as an adult). When you were faced with challenges that made you anxious or depressed, you may have been expected to just suck it up, deal with life, and move on. However, we now know this is not a healthy way to cope.

A mental health stigma —a negative perception of those with mental health issues—is prevalent in many cultures, including our own. However, mental health was talked about more openly during and after the COVID pandemic since so many people were isolated and sharing their anxieties. Some people are more comfortable now talking about their mental health issues, although the majority are still not.

The state of mental healthcare today

Like primary care providers, there is a shortage of behavioral health providers. Not every health system does mental and behavioral health well. Some healthcare systems only offer 15 minutes of support. Others offer 30 minutes. The average time covered by commercial insurance is

45 minutes. Depending on the provider, visits may be offered in person, through video conferences (telemedicine), or on the phone.

Where I work, video visits are limited. In-person or telephone appointments are limited to 30 minutes or less. Many people do not find therapy engaging when they are speaking with someone over the phone, particularly when they haven't met the provider in person and distrust healthcare and/or mental health care. While there are many online ways of getting mental health, these services are not always covered by insurance and many people cannot afford to pay for therapy themselves. The mental healthcare system, much like traditional healthcare, is broken. In an ideal world, traditional and mental health would be worked on together.

Finding the right provider

I think finding a mental health provider is like dating. You want someone who specializes in the issue you have. Let me explain. If you suffer from excessive worry and anxiety, you want someone who specializes in anxiety. If you experienced trauma at any point in your life, you want a therapist who specializes in trauma (not all therapists do). If you have depression, you want someone who treats depression.

Mental healthcare is not a one size fits all proposition. In fact, it is the opposite—it is unique to each person and the success of care depends on both the personality of the provider and the relationship of trust they establish with their patients. Bad News Barbara is back with a reality check: most facilities do not offer specialized mental health care. Too many patients can't find a provider they connect well with and are left feeling disappointed, often never to return to mental health therapy when they need it the most, to heal and move forward with life. Many telehealth and telehealth video behavioral health services allow you to select your behavioral health provider based on your needs and their expertise. If you don't like the first provider assigned to you, you can try another. But this service is often limited to people who can afford to pay out of pocket or who have generous health insurance plans.

If you are in need of a mental health provider, contact your health insurance directly or through your employer, Medicaid, or Medicare to see what services are available to you. You may also have luck finding one online, through: https://www.samhsa.gov/find-help. (This link will also be in the resources section)

Types of mental health providers

Like in traditional healthcare, there are many behavioral health providers: Licensed Professional Counselor (LPC), Licensed Clinical Professional Counselor (LCPC), Licensed Clinical Social Worker (LCSW), Marriage and Family Counselor (MFC), Psychiatric APRN, Doctor of Psychology (PsyD), and MD Psychiatrist.

Most MD psychiatrists evaluate, diagnose, and prescribe medication and do not do therapy. Most other practitioners provide the therapy but do not prescribe medication. The level of education and title does not necessarily indicate the level of care you receive. As I mentioned before, each person is unique and where a specific provider may work for one person, they may not work for another.

If your PCP does a screening tool for general anxiety disorder (GAD-2, GAD-7) or depression (PHQ-2, PHQ-9) and they feel you would benefit from behavioral health care based on your symptoms, conversation, and their assessment of your mental health needs, you will be given a referral to a mental health provider. But that isn't a guarantee you'll get to see one quickly. Know there is a long wait time to get a behavioral health appointment. If needed, your PCP can prescribe medication if, through shared decision-making, you both determine it's the best course of action for you.

Some PCPs will prescribe medication without requiring therapy but often it is important to process the causes of your mental health issues with an expert and find new ways of coping. Life gets more complicated as we get older because there are more issues to deal with.

If you are seeing a non-psychiatric therapist who does not prescribe medication, you can give your consent (sign a medical release form) for your therapist to speak with your PCP and have your PCP prescribe the medication.

If you need anti-psychotic medication for your condition, you will be referred to a psychiatrist and they will most likely be the ones to prescribe these specialized medications. In an emergency situation, you may be seen by a psychiatrist in the ER for medication.

Therapy is hard. If you have been in therapy, you know what I mean. Reliving past experiences and learning to think and cope in a different way is hard. But if you do the work, you give yourself a better chance of improving your overall health and wellbeing.

For more information, mental health resources are provided in the resources section.

Supporting your own emotional well-being

I argue that life is more difficult for women—we must encounter so many more barriers than men (many of our barriers are created by men and we live in a society that values men over women). Not to mention, most childrearing responsibilities still lie with women. We also must juggle many things at the same time. Even women with the highest means are often responsible for household chores and child rearing.[21] What often happens? Your emotional well-being suffers. You cannot be everything to everyone all at once when there is no "me time" in your day.

Regardless of your gender—men have their share of challenges too–life can be hard. We do not give ourselves enough credit for how strong we are. Mindfulness and meditation can be important tools in coping with our challenges. These methods help us to focus on the present, let go of the past and not worry so much about the future.

Many people have been credited for this quote: "Yesterday is history. Tomorrow is a mystery. But today is a gift, and that is why it's called the present."

Taking time for meditation, prayer, or engaging in spirituality practices is important for the mind body connection. This is not new age philosophy. I have shown you that everything in your world affects your emotional and physical health. Sitting in silence alone with our thoughts can be uncomfortable, especially when beginning a mindfulness practice. But training your mind to focus on the present will have a positive impact on all aspects of your life.

You are where you are today because of everything that has happened to you up until this moment. You wouldn't be reading this book if you were not curious about how to get better health care than you've experienced for yourself or family members in the healthcare system. I take about 15 minutes every morning to meditate. I have tried many apps, and after viewing the Headspace's guide to meditation series on Netflix, Headspace is my meditation/mindfulness app of choice. If you have a Netflix account, check out the Headspace series. There is also a series for sleep. Sometimes, my mind is focused; other times, I finish the morning meditation and tell myself, "That didn't go well; maybe I'll try that again." I like starting my day with a bit of calm. I am not good at using the app during the day when I probably need it most, but I use it every night to calm my racing mind so I can sleep.

Patient Story

I met Mary only once. She came to see me for an annual woman's wellness exam. She was overdue for her pap smear, and due for multiple screenings. She was 41. Her health record was incomplete and while we were reviewing it together, she shared with me her traumatic childhood and adulthood. She was working a full-time job with benefits, in recovery, living alone, not in a relationship. The fact that she was sitting before me was a miracle. I would like to say that Mary's experience is unique, but unfortunately, I have met many women who have had to overcome many challenges in their lives beginning in childhood. These women are warriors. I asked Mary how she made it through those challenges and hurt and she looked me straight in the eyes and told me "I shook that shit out!" That has become my mantra when I find myself getting caught up in my past. It is not so easy to forget the past. But the past is behind us, there is nothing we can do about it but process what happened, focus on the present and dream for where we want our future paths to go.

Chapter Sixteen

———

Eat. Move. Rest. Repeat.

We have complicated the idea of living a healthy lifestyle. Influencers and companies are trying to sell us a wide range of products to make us healthy (if you look at the data, the companies and influencers are getting rich while the rest of us are getting sick). We must get back to the basics and simplify our lives.

When I talk to my patients about their health and how to improve their wellness, the most common response I get is "I am going to go to the gym."

Movement is essential, and I will speak to this at length, but I would argue that movement is only one component of a healthy lifestyle. A good balance of healthy eating, movement, and sleeping is critical for good physical and mental health.

The next three chapters go into greater detail on how to develop and sustain healthy eating, exercise, and sleeping habits. If you're not in perfect health, you may need to unlearn some habits and replace them with others. **Changing your behavior and attitude towards health and wellness may save you from living a life dependent on medications and machines for preventable disease.** It will also help you reach your life expectancy.

It takes about 30 days to make or break a habit. While results may not be immediate, committing to healthy eating, exercise, and sleep routines can transform your life. Just think. Thirty days to readjust a habit could lead to a lifetime of good health! A lifetime where you aren't spending a large part of your paycheck on medical bills and support services. A lifetime of working, going out with friends, playing with your babies and grandbabies, traveling, and embracing the best of what life can offer.

You don't have to do this work alone. I think—and research backs me up on this—it's important to create your own support communities to help with lifestyle changes. Maybe it is your family, a friend or a co-worker, a neighbor, someone at church or at your children's school. If you do not have anyone willing to support you, you can search Facebook and other online support websites for groups you can join for virtual support. In fact, some of these likeminded groups are extremely effective since you can share your experiences with others going through the same challenges you are.

The first step toward healthy living is making the commitment to change.

Chapter Seventeen

Eat

According to the Merriam-Webster dictionary, food is "material consisting essentially of protein, carbohydrate, and fat used in the body of an organism to sustain growth, repair, and vital processes and to furnish energy."

My health philosophy is pretty simple: If you eat crap, you feel like crap, and you can't crap!

When you eat good food in the right amounts, you feel good! When you eat bad food, you feel bad. People often find comfort in food but often their food choices (a large bowl of mac and cheese, pizza, chips, bread, chocolate, ice cream, cookies—you name it) make you feel even worse afterwards, not providing comfort in the long run. In this section, I want to help you understand how food affects your body and how you can use it to support good health.

What you put inside your body is just as important, if not more important, than how you use your body. We're always looking for quick fixes: fad diets, abdominal binders to shrink belly fat, medications, and surgeries. These may work in the short term, but for most, not in the long term.

Weight management plays a vital role in your overall health. Weight gain occurs when you consume more calories than you burn. On average, you should consume about 2000 calories per day to maintain your current weight. Height, age, gender, and whether you are trying to gain or lose weight are factors that affect your optimum consumption. But this is a nice round number to work with. I am not one to count calories, I think it is time-consuming and can be frustrating. But it can be useful to think back to yesterday, write down the things you ate and drank and look up the calorie content of each item online. Add those calories up. Then go back and look at what you did yesterday. Were you on your feet and active? Were you sitting all day at your desk, in a car, or on a sofa? Were you sleeping? You can also find online calculators that tell you how many calories you burned based on your activities.

Subtract the number of calories you burned from the number of calories you ate and see how close it comes to 2,000 calories. This exercise can help you see how quickly excess calories can add up and how easy it is to gain weight (for most people). Your weight will continue to go up if you do nothing to reduce the excess calories you consume.

There is no quick fix to weight loss

If you are tempted to give into the weight loss medication fad, think twice. The media makes it look like a magic bullet that takes all the work out of dieting. But, did you know that the average person only loses 14.9% of their body weight over 68 weeks.[22] To put this in context, someone taking a weight loss injectable who weighed 250 pounds would lose approximately 37 pounds over 1 year and 4 months. What?!! You pay about $1,000 per month for over a year and you're still overweight? This is only one study, but others out there show similar results, some with even less weight loss.

In contrast, by changing what you eat, moving and sleeping more, you can lose one to two pounds per week. That is 52 to 104 pounds in one year! And while you do this, you are developing new lifestyle habits that you can use throughout your life, without the possible side effects and high price tag of medication or the risks of surgery. That is not to say that some of you may not need more support to make lifestyle changes. Medication and surgery may be necessary based on how much weight you need to lose and your health conditions. You should know that, given the health risks of obesity, your insurance is required to cover nutrition counseling if you are obese.

Solid food, of course, isn't the only thing you might need to change. What you drink also affects your weight and health. Water, tea (without sugar), and black coffee (without sugar or cream) come from nature and have no calories. Water is essential to keep you hydrated. You should be drinking eight to ten glasses of water a day. Coffee and tea (green tea especially) decrease inflammation and in moderate quantities are good for your health. Most other things you might drink—sugary drinks, soda/pop, fruit juice (yes, even the juices that are marked as healthy are loaded with sugar), energy drinks, and milk—all have calories due to their high sugar content. The more of these you consume, the more calories you add to your daily diet. Some people consume as many calories in liquid form as they do from solid food. Water has zero calories. If you do not like water, add frozen fruit or slices of lemon, lime, or cucumber to it for natural flavoring. And invest in a water filter for the healthiest water possible. Avoid bottled water whenever you can, given the forever chemicals in the plastic that also increase health risks.

The type and quality of food you eat matters

We need to eat to live. Without food we die. But many of the foods marketed to us, and that too many of us prefer over what Mother Nature gives us in pure form, are also killing us. I want you to consider what "food" you are putting into your body. Think back to yesterday. From the time you woke to the time you went to bed, what exactly did you eat and drink?

Food is a funny thing. It gives us energy to live and grow, but it can also be harmful. Foods that come from a farm or field are good for you.

Vegetables, fruits, legumes, beans, nuts, and even fresh dairy and some meat are generally the best choice for you and your body.

But many foods we eat aren't even real food. They're not grown in nature but made in laboratories or in food manufacturing sites, packaged in plastic, and sent to sit on grocery store shelves for sometimes months at a time. Go into your cupboards, fridge, or freezer and look at any of the foods that came prepackaged. They could be pasta, canned soups, cookies, crackers, cereals, premade meals like macaroni and cheese, frozen breakfast sandwiches, waffles, pancakes, and frozen pizza. Look at the ingredient list and see how long it is and how many ingredients you can even pronounce. Then do an Internet search to see the harmful effects of some of these unpronounceable preservatives and flavorings as well as the forever chemicals and pesticides used in commercial farming.

I know some of you skeptics are going to say there are pesticides used in commercial produce farming and feed additives, pesticides, and herbicides used to raise livestock, and yes that's true. There are also health concerns about genetically modified (GMO) produce. Even some organic foods have pesticides and chemicals, since the wind can move these chemicals across commercial fields to organic farms. As we've moved away from an agricultural society to a heavily urban one, we have had to depend on others to feed us. Even if we only shop at farmers markets, we don't have complete control over the fresh foods we buy. But buying fresh single-ingredient food is still healthier for us than buying processed food. And that includes plant-based proteins that are made to imitate meat. They are still overly processed and have a lot of chemicals that our bodies don't need.

A word about organic. In the U.S., foods that have the label "USDA Organic" have to meet strict standards set by the US Department of Agriculture. Farmers can't farm with synthetic pesticides, fertilizers, genetically modified seeds, or sewage sludge. They can't give antibiotics or growth hormones to livestock. Food manufacturers that label processed foods as organic can't use artificial flavors, colors, or preservatives. Organic foods can't use radiation to kill germs. There is general agreement that certified organic foods offer slightly more nutrients with less artificial chemicals than conventionally farmed food. However, there is not enough scientific data to determine how much better these foods are for you. Because organic produce is often more expensive than non-organic produce, you might not be able to afford it anyway. That's okay. You can still get major benefits from eating fresh whole food. I do not buy organic labeled produce in the supermarket unless it is the same price or cheaper than the non-organic.

What you eat affects how you feel

If you're not convinced that what you eat matters, consider food from a different perspective. Think about the last meal you ate, how you felt while you were eating the food, and how you felt afterwards. I'm going to bet that if you had a meal that didn't contain many vegetables or plant-based foods, you probably felt tired afterwards. Maybe it was an hour afterwards, maybe it was several hours afterwards, but you probably felt like you needed a nap. And then what happened? Because the meal was probably so low in nutrients, your body used what little nutrients it had, stored the rest of the calories as fat, and then signaled to your brain that it was hungry again as it searched for sufficient nutrients.

However, if you had a meal that included a large serving of steamed, sauteed, or raw vegetables, I suspect you felt pretty good after that meal. And what I mean by feeling good is that you felt like you had more energy and were not hungry again for several hours—until it was time for another meal.

146

Food for our bodies is like gasoline we put into our cars. Whenever we need to fill the gas tank, we make sure to put the correct type of gas into our cars. If not, we would ruin the engine. Why aren't we treating our bodies the same way? Our bodies should outlive our cars.

Stop thinking of "diet" as a verb

There is a difference between the word "diet" and the action "to diet." Diet is the sum total of what we eat and drink. "To diet" means to place restrictions on our eating, something that is hard to sustain over time without developing a kind of eating disorder. Dieting is all about fad diets.

When you deprive yourself of the foods you love over the long run, that deprivation can lead to binging when you finally reintroduce those beloved foods to your diet. If you ever did a low carb or keto diet, you know what I mean. Our bodies need carbohydrates (carbs), but carbs that come in the form of whole foods as I mentioned, not something neatly packaged with an attractive food label that was made in a factory.

To simplify meal prep and eating, I encourage you to use the diagram at the end of the last chapter. **Fill half your plate with vegetables, a quarter with nuts, seeds, whole grains, beans, and fruit, and the last quarter with a small portion of whatever else you want.** This could be meat, fish, cheese, or something else you love that isn't processed food. You don't have to measure out portions or calories. Simply use your plate as a guide for how much of each food to eat.

Why use 1/4 of your plate for whatever you want to eat? I learned this from Daphne Miller MD, a physician at the University of California San Francisco, who is an advocate for health equity and good farming practices. She recommends that 1/3 of the meal can be whatever her patients want. I am not great at math and think it's easier to divide the plate into 4 portions.

Also, to avoid binging, everyone is entitled to a cheat day, or shoot, even a cheat weekend or vacation. But if you do eat processed foods or food heavy in saturated fats or sugar, readjust and get back on your healthy-eating horse. Every day is a new opportunity to have a fresh start. You will notice that you feel better when you eat better, and those cheat days or meals become less frequent because you don't like the way you feel afterwards.

13 tips for Healthy Eating

If you're ready to give your body the fuel you need to live your best life, the following 13 tips are designed to help you rethink your relationship with food and build healthier eating habits that last.

1. Crack the code for healthy grocery shopping

Food companies have done an incredibly wonderful job of convincing us that we should eat their products, using colorful packaging and persuasive descriptions. But the next time you go grocery shopping, spend some time considering what you are really buying and whether it is food that provides the nutrients you need to thrive. Use the layout of the store to help you shop smartly.

In a traditional grocery store, the items that are on the perimeter (on the outer aisles of the store) are what you should eat more of: fresh produce, meat, seafood, and dairy. Generally, the produce section comes first, with its fresh fruits and vegetables. Vegetables could be celery, zucchini, eggplant, tomatoes, potatoes, onions, mushrooms, lettuce, spinach, asparagus. **One word to describe each food.** You get my drift. Fruits could be apples, oranges, lemons, limes, an array of berries like strawberries, blueberries, raspberries, pineapple, bananas, and mangoes. Sometimes across the aisle from the vegetable bins, you'll also find bulk grains, nuts, flour, and dried fruits. Also, one-word food items.

Then you'll have a refrigerated section with meat, seafood, dairy and eggs, which may be at the back of the store. In this section, you find steaks, pork chops, pork loin, lamb chops, chicken breast, chicken thighs, turkey breasts, salmon, cod, and catfish. The same pattern applies: **one, maybe 2, words describe that food.** Next comes dairy and eggs—cheese, yogurt, sour cream, milk. For the most part, what all these sections have in common is that they are real foods that come from nature. Some meats like sausages, hot dogs, lunch meats, and cheese, are processed, but their main ingredients came from animals. The dairy section is a little bit more convoluted, because there's a lot of other dairy-based products that are processed and have a lot of other chemicals that our bodies don't need (think Velveeta).

One side of a large grocery store frequently features fresh bakery goods and a deli counter. These foods are generally made fresh daily and don't have an ingredients list. Some can be healthy and others may be full of sugars and fats but without harmful preservatives.

All the middle aisles of the grocery store contain everything else, the prepackaged and frozen foods that are highly processed, created in large factories under sterile conditions, with multiple ingredients you probably cannot pronounce. If the freezer section is in a center aisle, it generally puts the fresh frozen vegetables, fruits, meats and fish (the foods that are better for you) closest to the outside aisle.

And why am I even going into this much detail? Because the food that Mother Nature provides gives us all the nutrients that our bodies need to function every day. So, if you limit your shopping to the outside perimeter of your grocery store, and resist the temptation of browsing the center aisles (as well as the bakery counter, which is often at the front of the store to promote impulse buying), you have the best chance of purchasing food that is healthy for you.

What about the supplement aisle, you might ask? It's usually one or two aisles in from the produce section, but that changes from store to store. There are physicians who market supplements under their own name, promising they will give our bodies exactly what they need. If physicians say we should take it, shouldn't we believe them? The issue is that supplements aren't regulated. People can slap a label on a package and tell you it's good for you even if it has not been scientifically proven to have a benefit. So, unless your healthcare provider has specifically prescribed a supplement because tests have determined you have a deficiency (such as iron) or are a vegetarian and need vitamin B12, spend your money on nutritious food. Here's the thing. Mother Nature has given us plenty of options that are packed with nutrients, neatly packaged and ready to eat on the go as well. You can take vegetables, fruit, seeds and nuts with you for nutritional support as easily as you can any supplement or energy bar.

2. Simplify your meals

When I talk to patients about their health risks, I often ask them to walk me through a typical day of meals and snacks. Often, they tell me it's too expensive, time-consuming, or difficult to eat healthy. They may say they don't know how to cook. But I'm here to show you that eating healthy can be affordable, quick, and easy—even if you're not a chef. A simple meal can take minutes to prepare, as the comparison below shows.

A Comparison of Two Meals:

Less healthy mac & cheese

>Boil water: 10 minutes

>Cook packaged pasta: 8 minutes

>Mix with butter and cheese: 1 minute

>Total prep time: 19 minutes

Healthy meal of veggies and protein

>Pan or air fry chicken breast: 10 minutes

>Microwave green beans: 5 minutes*

>Total prep time: 10 minutes

>*You can cook veggies while you cook your meat or fish.

Soon after you eat your big bowl of cheese and pasta meal, you are ready for a nap. After the chicken and green beans, you may have energy for a walk.

3. Prioritize vegetables

Mother Nature cannot make it easier for us. When you fill half your plate with vegetables, you get a meal packed with essential vitamins, minerals, and antioxidant – powerful compounds that protect your cells from damage. Since vegetables are low in calories, you can eat a whole plate's worth and consume less calories than you would with a small serving of pasta. Vegetables are high in fiber—which increases good cholesterol and decreases bad cholesterol. They are low in carbohydrates (there are carbs in vegetables, but they are rich in the nutrients our bodies need, easier to digest and better for us than the carbs in processed foods or foods with added sugars). Large portions of vegetables make you feel full sooner, and keep you satisfied for longer. Plus, vegetables are more affordable than many processed foods.

No matter how you buy your vegetables—fresh, frozen, or canned—they are equally nutritious, despite what you may see in the media. (If canned, buy the low sodium option or rinse them to remove the high salt content. Our bodies need salt but not that much.) Vegetables are quick to cook, and most can be eaten raw. Some vegetables, like potatoes and corn, get a bad rap for being high in carbs, but they are good for you, especially if eaten whole (keep the skin on potatoes because the skins are loaded with fiber, plus peeling the skin takes time).

Patients often tell me that they do not like vegetables and after further discussion, it is because they have never tried that many varieties or were given overcooked vegetables as children.

You can chop up raw or steamed vegetables and mix them with lettuce and beans or meat to make a salad, all in the matter of minutes. For an easy side dish, chop up cucumbers and red onion, mix, and sprinkle it with some vinegar and olive oil. You can also grab a bag of frozen stir fry vegetables and sauté them with strips of chicken breast. And again, dinner in minutes! If you want a quick snack, slice carrots, celery, radishes, or cucumbers and dip them in ranch dressing or hummus. While a lot of ranch dressing isn't great for you, if dipping your vegetables into it makes the vegetables taste better, then go ahead. Your body will thank you. Meal prep can really be that simple.

When buying fresh vegetables, it is always less expensive to purchase whatever is in season. For example, zucchini and yellow squash in the summer, butternut and acorn squash in the fall. If you are able, buy at your local farmer's market. The vegetables will taste better and support local farms rather than big corporations. Many farmer's markets accept SNAP Benefits. Another option is to subscribe to a farm box service that delivers a box of fresh vegetables to your door weekly, or as often as you like. The most affordable subscription services offer "imperfect" produce that grocery stores won't sell because it doesn't look beautiful. But everything in the box is as nutritious and delicious once peeled, cut, and or cooked. Check online for farm box delivery services.

If access to produce is an issue for you and you're worried that fresh vegetables will spoil before you can eat them all, stock up on frozen and canned vegetables when you go to the grocery store, especially when they're on sale. If you want to try new vegetables but don't want to spend money on those you're not sure you'll like, get together with family or friends, have each buy a different vegetable, prepare it, and share it in one meal. This is a very inexpensive way to try new things. Another cheap way to try different vegetables is to find a grocery store with a salad bar, put a few different vegetables in your box, and take them home and try them raw or cooked.

The staples I always have at home are golden potatoes, carrots (not the baby kind, whole), baby spinach, onions, frozen mixed vegetables, peas, broccoli, corn, mixed berries, canned tomatoes, black and red beans, tuna and salmon (for my husband, not for me, because I am a vegetarian), olive oil, nuts, and ground coffee.

4. Eat fruit wisely

Did you notice I have not yet mentioned fruit? We are programmed from an early age to prefer sweet flavors. But fruit is expensive and if fruit is your version of healthy food, I would understand if you told me you cannot afford to eat healthy. But that is not my advice. Your portion of fruit should be small, less than 1/4 of your plate when you divide your plate into four sections. When I was growing up, fruit was a treat, often eaten for dessert and only eaten when in season. I recommend you put it in that same special treat category.

Frozen fruit is a less expensive option and a good choice for adding fruit to your diet. Make sure you buy fresh frozen fruit with no added sugar. If you do not have time to prepare a meal, and you have a blender (I am shocked by how many of my patients have blenders but don't use them), you can combine a small amount of frozen fruit along with vegetables (think spinach, kale, cucumbers, celery) and water to create a green smoothie with some sweetness. This gives you multiple servings of vegetables that you can make and drink quickly. If you want more nutrients, add flax or chia seeds. Better to drink the smoothie straight away rather than take it with you, because the nutrients break down over time.

Juicers that extract all fiber and make a clear colored liquid are a waste of money and contribute to food waste. You and your body need that extracted fiber. Regular juicing is actually very expensive because you need large quantities of vegetables and fruit to make a small glass of juice. (Plus, those machines are huge and take up a lot of counter space.) Keep things simple. Chuck everything in a blender, add water, blend and drink.

5. Get fiber and protein from whole grains, beans, nuts, and seeds

Beans, peas, lentils, soy (tofu), nuts, seeds, and whole grains (quinoa, buckwheat, farro, wheat berries, oats, rice) are rich in fiber and nutrients, many are high in protein, and most are inexpensive.

Protein is an essential nutrient vital for every part of your body. Often called the "building blocks" of life, protein is involved in the structure, function, and regulation of tissues and cells. There are thousands of different proteins, each with a specific job.

Proteins are made up of chains of amino acids. While there are 20 amino acids, nine are essential, meaning your body can't produce them. **You must get these essential amino acids from the foods you eat.** Combining grains like rice with legumes such as beans or lentils creates a complete protein. This pairing provides all the essential amino acids your body needs

Fiber is a nutritional powerhouse. It helps regulate digestion, keeps you feeling full, and can lower your risk of heart disease, diabetes, and certain cancers. Found exclusively in plants, fiber is abundant in whole grains, beans, nuts, and seeds.

There is debate about brown rice versus white rice. Both are naturally grown, though white rice, which is refined, offers fewer nutrients because the bran and germ of the grain have been stripped away. In many parts of the world where people live well past life expectancy—like Okinawa, Japan and Costa Rica—white rice is eaten in small quantities. When considering rice versus pasta for a meal, rice is the better choice. If you want to add beans to a meal but don't have time to soak and cook dry beans, canned beans are a good option. But if you have high blood pressure and salt is an issue, buy low sodium beans and rinse them before heating them or adding them to a salad.

6. Embrace healthy fats

A word about fats. Just like carbohydrates and proteins, our bodies need healthy fats to function properly. The key is understanding the difference between good fats and bad fats.

The Mediterranean diet, known for its health benefits, is a great example. It emphasizes good fats like olive oil, olives, fish, nuts, and even avocados (good for brain health). You can add these fats to your meals by using small amounts of olive oil for pan-frying meat or fish, or by drizzling it on vegetables and salads.

While the debate about which oils are the best for you, research suggests plant-based oils are generally a better choice. When adding oil to any meal, moderation is key – the less oil you use, the better.

Also, be cautious of certain diets, like keto, that promote unrestricted fat intake. Some fats, particularly unsaturated fats from animal sources (excluding fish), are not good for you in high quantities.

7. Moderate your meat intake

People have been eating meat since they learned to kill animals. If you are a vegetarian, I get it, so am I. But most people eat meat. Too much of it. Reducing your portion size of meat can help lower your intake of saturated fat and cholesterol, both of which can contribute to heart disease. Meat provides protein, which you need to be healthy. On average, women need around 46 grams of protein a day and men need an around 56 grams. If you don't follow a strictly plant-based diet but do follow the guidelines for vegetables, beans, grains and seeds, you need less than one 5- to 8-ounce portion of beef, chicken or pork a day to fulfill your protein intake.

Red meat (beef) is not essential to a healthy diet. In fact, recent data suggest that the average U.S. resident eats over 83 pounds of beef a year, way over the global average of 20 pounds[23] and above dietary guidelines. Eating excessive amounts of beef has been shown to contribute to the sad fact that someone in the U.S. dies every 33 seconds from cardiovascular disease.[24] While red meat does provide protein, iron, and zinc, these nutrients can be obtained from other sources like beans, lentils, and tofu.

Leaner meat options like chicken and turkey without skin are good sources of protein with lower fat content.

Beyond its contribution to heart disease, **let's talk about the real problem with meat.** The real problem is how badly animals are raised (not as nature intended), how they are killed, and how the people who process the animals are treated. Meat farming is factory farming, big business subsidized by the federal government. Whenever there is a hurricane or fire, you read how thousands, even millions of animals died. That's because they were confined to small spaces and were trapped inside. We often do not care where are meat comes from, as long as we can get it and get it cheap. But, if you are a meat eater, the way animals are raised and killed (stressed from birth to death, often pumped up with hormones) has a big impact on your health because you are eating the animal's stress and hormones.

The same holds true for the egg debate. Eggs are incredibly nutritious and affordable. Some may even argue an egg is the perfect food. But people freak out when egg prices climb. I want you to look at it from a different perspective. When you buy from a supplier that raises healthy free-range chickens that lay healthy eggs, like Vital Farms, the price for a dozen eggs may be as high as $9.00. But if eggs are the protein for your main meal and you eat 2 per day, you are spending only $1.50 for that portion of that meal. Significantly less than a Big Mac.

There are ways to raise animals that are healthy for human consumption. Animals raised humanely are less stressed, leaner and better for us. If you're going to eat meat, make it a special occasion and spend a little more for the sake of your and the animal's health! If you have the luxury, shop for meat at a butcher that you know sources pasture-raised meat. To say I am a huge fan of Costco is an understatement. They are a company that cares about where their products come from and have made strides in animal welfare standards so the quality of their meat is higher than many other stores.

To learn more about meat farming and production, check out the Resource section at the end of the book.

8. Add fatty fish to your diet.

Fish is a fantastic source of lean protein, essential fatty acids, and various vitamins and minerals. Omega-3 fatty acids, found abundantly in fatty fish such as salmon, mackerel, and sardines, are particularly good for heart health. These nutrients help lower blood pressure, reduce inflammation, and decrease the risk of heart disease. To reap these rewards, aim to eat at least two servings of fish per week.

9. Stick with real food

Many companies are trying to sell you meat alternatives—not-dogs, not-burgers, tofurkey— but these items are also highly processed and often cost more than the real thing! What! The plant-based meat alternatives cost more than meat?

There is no substitute for real whole food. You want a burger, then eat a beef, chicken, or turkey burger. You want something plant-based, then eat plants. If you love veggie burgers, there are many recipes that use a range of different vegetables, beans and grains that are easy and quick to make.

By eating whole food, you can make small changes in the healthcare system and in the food system.

10. Enhance the flavor of food with herbs and spices

Herbs and spices are the secret to making your food taste better. These flavorful additions not only enhance taste but also add depth and complexity to your meals, transforming simple ingredients into extraordinary flavors. Add herbs like oregano, basil, parsley, cilantro, thyme, and rosemary to vegetables, meats, and salads. Spices like pepper, paprika, cumin, chili powder, cayenne, and turmeric all are great staples to keep in your spice drawer to elevate a sauce, soup or egg dish.

11. Make healthier versions of your favorite foods

Think of your favorite foods. Nearly all of them can be made healthier. I have a large Latina population and corn tortillas and arepas are staples. Traditionally, tortillas were made by soaking corn in lime juice and water, then pounding this mixture to make a dough, forming the dough into balls, flattening them by hand, cooking them on a comal, and eating them immediately. There is no shelf life to making tortillas this way. They harden if not eaten straight away. That's why store-bought tortillas have preservatives.

Tortillas were designed to hold food. But the cheese, meat, or veggies you place inside a tortilla can be eaten alone or placed inside a cabbage or lettuce leaf for a healthier option. If you miss the flavor of the corn, keep a bag of corn in your freezer, defrost and throw it on the comal or cast-iron skillet on dry heat. Then add it to the filling you would otherwise put in a tortilla. You get a charred flavor, and you are eating a whole food—vegetable rather than the store-bought tortillas that last forever. Corn can be a substitute for corn bread. And you'll find some of the corn in the toilet the next day and know that the fiber in the corn did its job cleaning your colon.

Love pizza? Take pizza sauce, mozzarella cheese, pepperoni or any toppings of your choice, place them on top of large tomato slices and bake or broil them. Or use the sauce, cheese and other goodies as a topping on a baked potato. You still get the flavor of the pizza without the carbs of the crust. Love macaroni and cheese. Make your cheese sauce (not the healthiest option) so you do not deprive yourself of your favorite food, and mix it with chopped cauliflower and/or potatoes with the skin on. You still get the flavor of the mac and cheese but without all the carbs and processed ingredients in macaroni.

There are so many places online where you can find healthy recipes based on any diet, cultural, and ethnic traditions. My philosophy is to start simple—create easy meals with a few ingredients. You want to enjoy cooking meals at home rather than rely on others to cook your meals. Unless you love to cook, it's best to forget complicated meals with many unknown ingredients that leave you frustrated and make you want to throw in the towel.

12. Invest in the right appliances

If you can, invest in some appliances that makes cooking easier. My best friend is the Instant Pot. I do not know where I would be in my life if I did not have it. I cook hard boiled eggs, rice, beans, lentils, steam vegetables, potatoes for potato salad or mashed potatoes, soups, chilis, sauces in my Instant Pot. I am not even using it to its fullest. Slow cookers (aka crockpots) are also a good investment, especially if you want to cook a roast or one dish meal that you prepare in the morning and have ready 8 hours later. Air Fryers cook meat and vegetables without using oil (you may need a little but not as much as you would if you fried something on the stove). Air fryers cook faster than baking something in the oven. Microwaves are great for steaming vegetables, reheating leftovers, and even cooking scrambled eggs. There are so many resources online for recipes using specific appliances and I am in awe and grateful for the people who post recipes specifically for these appliances, because they have made my life easier!

13. Create a meal plan

BARBARA'S DAILY INSTRUCTIONS FOR A HEALTHY LIFE

Create a weekly meal plan based on your favorite foods, online recipe searches, or a simple cookbook. Create a grocery list from the menu. Make sure you are grocery shopping on a full stomach so you aren't tempted to buy items that are not on your list (and not good for you). Create a pantry of go-to staples. Most vegetables and whole grains, beans, nuts and seeds are shelf stable, meaning they will last longer if properly stored. Doing your meal planning and grocery shopping weekly puts all the ingredients on hand to prepare your own meals.

Your sample meal plan

To jumpstart your health eating program, here are a few sample menus based on my plate recommendations. At the beginning of the week, prep food by washing fresh vegetables so they are ready to cut up and add to each recipe. Also, boil 12 eggs to eat for breakfast or have for lunch in a salad.

Breakfast	Lunch	Dinner
Grits with sauteed spinach, mushrooms, zucchini and onions	Cabbage leaf wraps with ground turkey, tomato, onion, topped with hot sauce a little mayonnaise	Roast with potatoes, carrots and onions
Piece of toast – you choose what type of bread	Apple with peanut butter	
Black coffee, tea or lemon water	Water, iced herbal tea	Water with a slice of cucumber

Breakfast	Lunch	Dinner
Two hard boiled eggs	Salad with chopped cucumbers, tomatoes, red or white onion, can of chickpeas drained and rinsed, black olives	Seasoned chicken breast (panfried, air fried or baked), make extra for lunch the next day.
Tomato slices seasoned with salt	Make a simple vinaigrette salad dressing from scratch (basically vinegar, Dijon mustard, olive oil, salt and pepper) that can be used on multiple salads	Frozen peas seasoned with salt, pepper, steamed in the microwave and served with a pat of butter
Chopped fruit		Can of white beans rinsed and heated up.
Black coffee, tea or lemon water	Water, iced herbal tea	Water with a slice of cucumber

Breakfast	Lunch	Dinner
Scrambled eggs with vegetables (onion, zucchini, and/or mushrooms)	Spinach salad with sliced cold chicken breast, red onion, apple slices and walnuts	Pork chop—pan or air fried, seasoned with salt and pepper
Small cup of fruit	Use the salad dressing you made the day before, mix all together	Mashed potatoes with the skin on
		Green beans (fresh or canned, cooked, seasoned with salt and pepper)
Black coffee, tea or lemon water	Water, iced herbal tea	Water

Breakfast	Lunch	Dinner
Spinach, cucumber, celery smoothie with frozen fruit, chia or flax seeds. Add water so it's not too thick.	Canned tuna salad lettuce wraps (make tuna salad with celery and onion, mayo, salt and pepper)	White fish seasoned with old Bay's seasoning
	Mixed nuts	Fresh or frozen broccoli
		Rice (make extra to have for dinner the next night)
Black coffee, tea or lemon water	Water, iced herbal tea	Water with a slice of cucumber

Breakfast	Lunch	Dinner
Spinach, cucumber, celery smoothie with frozen fruit, chia or flax seeds. Add water so it's not too thick.	Egg salad lettuce cups (make an egg salad with hardboiled eggs, place inside lettuce leaves	Chicken breast thinly sliced
	Mixed nuts	Frozen stir fry vegetables cooked in peanut oil or canola oil, splashes of low sodium soy sauce
		rice
Black coffee, tea or lemon water	Water, iced herbal tea	Water

Chapter Eighteen

Move

Movement helps reduce stress levels and break up the monotony in our days. Movement also helps you sleep better. And the more you move, the more energy you have, and the better you feel.

Sitting has become the new smoking. Years ago, smoking was a leading cause of death. While cigarette use has decreased, sitting for prolonged periods of time (especially at a computer or in front of a screen) has increased. I always ask my patients what kind of activity they do daily. The most common response is "not much."

The good news is that increasing your activity doesn't not have to involve going to a gym. Any kind of movement on a daily basis is going to have positive health benefits.

Children used to play out in the streets and occupied their time with different forms of play, always on the move. Now playtime has been replaced with sitting down watching a television screen or tablet, playing video games, or texting or talking on the phone. As children grow up today, they don't miss movement because it was never a big part of their lives.

I recognize that many people do not have access to safe places to play or move outside. Our communities have not done a good job of investing in recreational areas, particularly in urban areas. Of course, environmental pollution has created other challenges, since in many places, being outside for prolonged periods of time is not healthy. This is particularly an issue for people who have asthma, a condition concentrated in underserved urban areas.

As adults, we've become more dependent on cars or public transportation to get from one place to another. For many, most of the time at work is spent sitting. As adults we are also spending time on our phones, streaming television shows or movies, and sitting rather than moving. Rather than going out shopping, which involves some walking around, you may have everything you buy delivered to your home. This lack of activity is negatively affecting our health and causing harm. We need to move more! (Some of you may just need to start moving).

For many people going to the gym is expensive. For others who are too busy to schedule a time to go to the gym, the thought is probably stressful. But finding ways in your day where you can incorporate more movement will make you feel better. Movement increases the happy hormones in our brains. Movement gives us more flexibility, helps us burn off calories, and is good for our bodies and overall health. For people who are diabetic or have high blood pressure, an increase in physical activity can improve health outcomes. In fact, studies show that people who are diabetic and are more active have better sugar control. They also show that people with arthritis have less pain when they are more active.

Exercise at home

There are so many ways where you can incorporate movement into your life. At home, regardless of your age, there are YouTube videos with exercise routines. You can subscribe to Zoom workout programs with live trainers, or dance to music videos. Dancing is a fabulous exercise that moves many body parts at the same time. There are many free apps online that make movement affordable.

Resistance training, especially after menopause and as you age, builds muscle, helps protect bones, and reduces fall risk and injury due to a fall. Resistance training is easy and free when you use your own body. Jumping jacks, wall sits, planks, high knees, running in place, squats, lunges, sit ups, and push-ups are all forms of resistance training. You can also use ankle or hand weights while walking to increase resistance and build muscles. Squats are a great exercise to support the muscles around the hips. If you are unable to do a full squat, support yourself by holding on to something or just sit down, stand up, sit down for 10 or more repetitions. Try to do resistance training 2 to 3 times per week, increasing the number of cycles you do each exercise.

I love the 7-minute workout. Johnson & Johnson pioneered a study about how to work every muscle in your body in 7 minutes. It has since been studied and is well validated.[25] Though their app is no longer available, there are other free 7-minute programs online that use the same form of high intensity interval training (HIIT). Basically, you do an exercise for 30 seconds, rest 10 seconds, and then do another exercise until you've covered 12 exercises or more. If you have more than 7 minutes, you can repeat the sequence. You can use the resistance training exercises mentioned above, lift weights, jump rope, or jump on a trampoline. You get a great workout in a short amount of time. The more intervals you can do, the better, but a good 7-minute session is a great start, especially if you don't think you have time to exercise.

Another option, if you're streaming television shows or movies, is to stand up, march in place, walk side to side, jog up and down, or do jumping jacks, squats, or lunges while you're watching your shows. You can get in a lot of exercise during a 30-minute episode and not miss what's happening on the screen. Or, if you're sitting down to watch the show, during the commercial break, get up and walk around the room or throughout your home. No commercials? Press pause every 20 minutes for 3 minutes and walk around. That's movement.

Another way to incorporate movement into your day is house cleaning. When you clean your house, you're using all different muscle groups:

squatting, bending, stretching, lifting, twisting. If your house is clean already, dance.

Exercise at work

If you drive to work, park further away, walk around the parking lot or walk around your building prior to starting work. Do the same thing on your lunch breaks. Eat lunch and then walk around for the remainder of your break. Do the same before getting into your car to go back home.

During your workday, you can set an alarm on a smart watch, your phone, or computer to remind you every hour to get up and move. The standard recommendation is to get up and move for two to five minutes every hour.

If you rely on public transportation, think about biking to work, if you can, or get off two stops earlier and walk the remainder of the way. Do the same on your way home. Get off a few stops ahead and get a walk in before calling it a day. If you work from home and your neighborhood allows, go for a 20- to 30-minute walk prior to starting your day. Think of it as your commute time. And do the same thing at the end of the day. You're incorporating more physical activity into your daily routine without having to do anything dramatically different, plus you will feel calmer starting and ending your day with that walk.

Find your fitness tribe

Early in 2024, I took a mental health leave of absence from work due to burnout. During this time, I signed up for self-defence classes. I thought if I could defend myself physically, I would be better at defending myself mentally. After I returned to work, I realized how much stronger and more confident I was after taking these classes. But I also realized how quickly I became part of a community, seeing the same people at class. I had a routine for exercise, but until I started participating, I didn't realize all the benefits of group classes. Group exercise is a great way to build a supportive community and reduce loneliness while also improving physical and mental health.

If you have family and friends who also want to live healthier lives, organize a walking group. You can walk in your neighborhood, on a school track, at a local mall, in a public park, or on bike or hiking trails. If you like riding a bike join a cycling group that bikes regularly.

If you have a community center, see if there are inexpensive group classes you can take or gym equipment you can use for free. If you can join a private gym or attend school where there are group classes, take advantage of that.

The truth is that there is always time for movement. But it takes discipline to get up and move when you've gotten used to sitting all day. Instead of focusing on the 7 minutes to an hour you might put into movement, focus on the way you'll feel when you get older and don't have any health conditions to limit what you can do with your life.

Chapter Nineteen

———

Rest

A lot of people think rest is overrated. I'm going to show you how wrong that attitude is.

Rest can be many things, but first let's talk about sleep. Sleep is important for our physical and mental health. It's easy to fall into the trap of thinking you have too many things to accomplish each day and can't afford to sacrifice productive hours for more sleep. But if you take inventory of your day, think how much time is wasted doing things that don't benefit your health and welfare.

That's not to say, that many people—and you may be one of them—work two or three jobs to make ends meet and don't have the luxury of resting as much as your body needs. It's also not unusual to work full time, return home to take care of your children and household chores, and feel you don't have an extra minute to breathe let alone sleep. I have many patients who are students in junior high, high school, and college who get very few hours of sleep because they stay up late studying.

But here's the thing, if you're sleep deprived, you may go through your day exhausted and are less efficient at getting any of your tasks completed effectively. If you're in school, you can't retain much of the information you're studying. So, the time you spend trying to accomplish too much is actually wasted.

The human body needs on average of seven hours of sleep a night (experts advise 7 to 9 hours of sleep each night). Both too much and too little can cause complications, including chronic disease in years to come. A recent study concluded that irregular sleep patterns can increase your risk of type 2 diabetes.[26] Research has also proven that staying awake for up to 19 hours without sleep is like functioning legally drunk.[27] It can impair your performance in multiple areas, including driving a car.

I know many of you reading this are saying to yourself you can function with four or five hours of sleep per night. But you can't. Not for prolonged periods of time. I've included a link to an article in resources section titled "How Drunk Are You Without Sleep? Check it out.

For those of you who are sleeping four or five hours a night, think about how you feel as you go through your day. Are you sluggish or irritable? Do you find yourself grabbing energy drinks, drinking lots of coffee, or eating to keep your energy levels up so you don't feel tired during the day? Do you find yourself losing focus or struggling to make decisions or solve problems? Are you more forgetful? These can be signs of being sleep deprived and if you don't change your behavior, lack of sleep will limit your quality of life. Your body needs to sleep to recuperate from the stress placed on it the day before.[28] Chronic lack of sleep also stresses your body so it cannot defend itself against illness like the common cold.

Create a bedtime routine

Going to bed at different hours every night (or day if you happen to work a nightshift) makes it hard to get a good night of sleep. It's important to create a bedtime routine so that you can get 7 hours of sleep each night (or day). Try to go to bed at roughly the same time and get up at the same time every day. Resist the temptation to go to bed late one night and then make up for it by sleeping in the next.

It's also important to create a good sleep environment. If your room is too hot, bright, or noisy, this can impact your sleep. If you bring technology into your bedroom, this can also make it hard to drift off easily. So many of us are addicted to our phones or screens that we can't seem to put them down once we start watching videos or surfing social media channels. Whatever you are streaming or looking at on social media, it won't suddenly disappear the next day. If it does, it wasn't that important.

If you can't avoid others in your bedroom using technology, invest in earplugs, a sleep mask, black out curtains, sound machines, or fans to create a better sleep environment so you can get the rest that you need.

A good mattress is also one of the best investments you can make in your health. You should be spending one third of your life in bed sleeping. Your sleep may suffer when you use an old mattress that doesn't give you support. This also applies to the size and number of pillows you use. If you're sleeping with a pillow that doesn't support your neck or too many pillows (head pillows and body pillows), you may not be getting a good night's sleep either because your spine is twisted or your neck improperly extended. Poor sleep posture not only affects your sleep but can increase pain from arthritis, making it hard to get through the day.

Some health conditions can also affect sleep quality. Pain, snoring, sleep apnea, or having a partner with these conditions can prevent you from getting the sleep you need. If the latter and earplugs don't work, sleep in a different room. You can still have sex with your partner, but probably not in the middle of the night. If you do sleep separately, however, you will be better rested and able to enjoy the waking time you have together.

Slow down the pace of your life

Rest isn't just about sleep. In this day and age our lives are over scheduled and finding a better balance provides a rest break from chaos. You may have a fear of missing out if you don't say yes to every activity or invitation —whether you are a parent and want your children to be involved in many extracurricular activities or you're afraid of missing a social event with your friends or family. At work, you may spend more time trying to get that promotion, working overtime, or finishing up all the tasks that have been assigned that cannot be done in an 8-hour shift. You need to know your limitations, make time for rest, and prioritize your health. If you don't, you may not be alive to enjoy everything you're working for.

Rest is also about playing. You need time for recess like you had as a child. You need time to play, no matter your age. It's a mental break from stress. And as adults, we forget what it means to play. If you are able, learn a new hobby, join a book club, play pickle ball or attend a Zumba class. Breaking up our routines is good for our mental health.

If you have a stressful job, a stressful home environment, or if you're juggling working and taking care of children, it's hard to find much time during the day to play. You may need to schedule an hour or two one day a week where you're left undisturbed. If you're working multiple jobs, find a way to schedule your shifts so you can get some time to yourself every week.

You may need to learn to say no to work and yes to rest and play to care for your physical and mental health.

Chapter Twenty

———

Repeat

Keep making the changes to the way you eat, move, and sleep until they are well established habits.

I wish I had a human hologram, like Princess Laia in Star Wars, to show my patients (and you) how possible it is to achieve a place of health and wellness. How simple it really can be to eat, move, and sleep in a healthier way and make this part of your lifestyle.

When I have a patient who has an appointment, and I see significant health improvements—weight loss, strength, healthy results on blood tests, a positive mood—I ask what motivated them to change their lifestyle. Most times I am told they were sick and tired of hearing me fuss on them. But when I ask how they feel, they will tell me they feel better, have more energy, and are more active.

I ask if they felt deprived by having to make major changes in their day-to-day activities and spend more money on food and the answer is always no. In fact, they are amazed how much money they are saving by eating healthier and preparing meals at home.

These moments make my heart sing and bring me joy. Changing habits and making new ones are difficult but doable. Your current lifestyle did not happen overnight, nor will creating a new one. It's easier to make bad habits than to break them. Have patience my friend. Start small. Choose one thing in each category (eat, move, rest, repeat) that you can do now, and build on your accomplishments.

While the healthcare system is designed to provide essential services, it's ultimately up to each of us to manage our own health. By forming healthy habits, making informed choices, and advocating for our needs, we can overcome the challenges posed by a system that does not always have our backs.

You are important. You are worth making the investment to achieve a state of good health and wellness, to live to a ripe old age. I believe in you.

Chapter Twenty-One

———

Resources

For convenient access to these electronic resources, please visit https://www.barbaraalifdoran.com.

List of questions to ask your provider

- Can I have an interpreter if one is not offered for you?
- Can we review my chart to make sure that everything is up to date?
- Should I be worried about anything in my chart that will affect my health in the future?
- I am worried about ...
- I am struggling with ...
- I need help with ...
- Why are you ordering these tests? Will I have to pay for the tests? Is this something my insurance will pay for?
- How will I know if my test results are normal? What do I do if they are abnormal?
- How can I communicate with you after my visit if I have any questions? Is there an app or a website where I can go to see my test results, ask questions or make a follow-up appointment?
- When do I need to make another appointment?

Where to find health information

MENTAL HEALTH

Mental Health Hotline/Crisis hotline

If you are in a crisis, or feel like you need to speak with someone, help is available 24/7 in English, Spanish and for the deaf/hearing impaired.

Dial 988. Keep this number under your favorites on your cell phone

https://988lifeline.org/?utm_source=google&utm_medium=web&utm_

For readers living outside the USA, click on the links below to find resources in your country.

Worldwide, many people have WhatsApp

https://faq.whatsapp.com/1417269125743673

Psychology Today: this is also a good resource to search specific behavioral healthcare providers

https://www.psychologytoday.com/us/basics/suicide/suicide-prevention-hotlines-resources-worldwide

DOMESTIC AND INTIMATE PARTNER VIOLENCE

Domestic Violence (Intimate Partner Violence) Hotline

Call 1-800-799-7233 or text "START" to 88788

TTY: 1-800-787-3224

You can also visit the National Domestic Violence Hotline's website and have a live chat

https://www.thehotline.org/?utm_source=youtube&utm_medium=organ

National Sexual Assault Hotline:

Call 1-800-656-HOPE; 1-800-656-4673

Or visit RAINN website to have a live chat and to learn more:

https://www.rainn.org[1]

For Teens experiencing dating violence:

Call 1-866-331-9474 or text LOVEIS to 22522

You can also visit the Love Is Respect website to have a live chat and find more information:

https://www.loveisrespect.org[2]

Strong Hearts Native Helpline:

Call 1-844-7NATIVE (762-8483).

Or visit their website for a live chat and to learn more:

https://strongheartshelpline.org[3]

Outside the USA:

Women Against Violence Europe

https://wave-network.org/list-of-helplines-in-46-countries/

Mystic Mag is helpful to find domestic violence resources worldwide

https://www.mysticmag.com/psychic-reading/domestic-violence-resource-guide/

---

1. https://www.rainn.org/

2. https://www.loveisrespect.org/

3. https://strongheartshelpline.org/

SUBSTANCE USE DISORDERS

SAMHSA - Substance Abuse and Mental Health Services Administration

The https://www.samhsa.gov/find-help/national-helpline.

What is SAMHSA's National Helpline?

SAMHSA's National Helpline, 1-800-662-HELP (4357) (also known as the Treatment Referral Routing Service), or TTY: 1-800-487-4889 is a confidential, free, 24-hour-a-day, 365-day-a-year, information service, in English and Spanish, for individuals and family members facing mental and/or substance use disorders. This service provides referrals to local treatment facilities, support groups, and community-based organizations.

Also visit the online treatment locator[4], or send your zip code via text message: 435748 (HELP4U) to find help near you. Read more about the HELP4U text messaging service[5].

CHRONIC HEALTH CONDITIONS

Diabetes information: The American Diabetes Association https://diabetes.org/?utm_source=google&utm_medium=paidsearch&ut totepremium&utm_content=responsive-search-ad&utm_term=geo&gclid=CjwKCAiA29auBhBxEiwAnKcSqqQPhF6_N MHOFEokIK_ROr_DCJBA2bBoCRaMQAvD_BwE

High blood pressure, heart disease.

The CDC https://www.cdc.gov/heartdisease/

The American Heart Association: https://www.heart.org/en/

---

4. https://findtreatment.samhsa.gov/

5. https://www.samhsa.gov/find-help/national-helpline/help4u

Signs and Symptoms of a heart attack or Stroke

Signs of Stroke in Men And Women
If any of the following signs appear suddenly, call 9-1-1 right away.

- Numbness or weakness in the face, arm, or leg, especially on one side of the body.
- Confusion or trouble speaking or understanding speech.
- Trouble seeing in one or both eyes.
- Trouble walking, dizziness, or problems with balance.
- Severe headache with no known cause.

Source: CDC https://www.cdc.gov/stroke/signs_symptoms.htm#:~:text=Sudden%20numbness%20or%20weakness%20[6].

Heart Attack
Signs and symptoms in women and men

- Chest pain or discomfort
- Shortness of breath
- Pain or discomfort in the jaw, neck, back, arm, or shoulder
- Feeling nauseous, light-headed or unusually tired

6. https://www.cdc.gov/stroke/signs_symptoms.htm

Source: CDC https://www.cdc.gov/heartdisease/heart_attack.htm

Cancer information:

Centers for Disease Control (CDC)

https://www.cdc.gov/cancer/

Cancer risk, prevention and screening:

https://www.cancer.org/research/acs-research-news/facts-and-figures-2024.html#[7]

https://www.cancer.gov[8]

https://www.who.int/news-room/fact-sheets/detail/cancer

Calculate my BMI (body mass index): Remember, the BMI gives you a ballpark idea of weight

The National Institutes of Health https://www.nhlbi.nih.gov/health/educational/lose_wt/BMI/bmicalc.htm

HEALTH INSURANCE

The Health Insurance Marketplace:

https://www.usa.gov/health-insurance-marketplace

Medicaid and Children's Health Insurance Program (CHIP)

https://www.healthcare.gov/medicaid-chip/

Specifically for CHIP

https://www.insurekidsnow.gov/coverage/index.html

---

7. https://www.cancer.org/research/acs-research-news/facts-and-figures-2024.html

8. https://www.cancer.gov/

Indian Health Service

https://www.ihs.gov/aboutihs/

https://www.ihs.gov/forpatients/

Find a Federally Qualified Health Center:

https://findahealthcenter.hrsa.gov[9]

Find discounted health insurance:

https://www.healthcare.gov/get-coverage/

DISCOUNT PRESCRIPTION DRUGS

Mark Cuban CostPlus Drug Company

https://costplusdrugs.com[10]

Good Rx

https://www.goodrx.com/drugs

Amazon Pharmacy for Prime Members

https://www.amazon.com/gp/help/customer/display.html?nodeId=T1RUrurdrUdeTYaRqp

Ask Walmart, Walgreen's or your local pharmacy about their prescription programs and whether you qualify for lower costs.

GENERAL HEALTH

Centers for Disease Control

https://www.cdc.gov[11]

---

9. https://findahealthcenter.hrsa.gov/

10. https://costplusdrugs.com/

The Mayo Clinic

https://www.mayoclinic.org/diseases-conditions

The Cleveland Clinic

https://my.clevelandclinic.org/health

The right to access your health record: The American Cures Act

https://www.healthit.gov/sites/default/files/page2/2020-03/
TheONCCuresActFinalRule.pdf

HEALTHY RECIPE RESOURCES

Well Plated by Erin

https://www.wellplated.com[12]

Two Sleevers

https://twosleevers.com[13]

Sweet Potato Soul

https://fitslowcookerqueen.com/about/

Hola Jalapeno

https://www.holajalapeno.com/about/

Jessica in the Kitchen

https://jessicainthekitchen.com[14]

Skinny Taste

https://www.skinnytaste.com[15]

I Heart Umami

https://iheartumami.com[16]

---

12. https://www.wellplated.com/
13. https://twosleevers.com/
14. https://jessicainthekitchen.com/
15. https://www.skinnytaste.com/
16. https://iheartumami.com/

FARMING AND ANIMAL WELFARE

Local independent farmers in your area and what they produce...

https://www.aspca.org/shopwithyourheart/consumer-resources/
shop-your-heart-grocery-list

Animal welfare issues

https://www.woah.org/en/what-we-do/animal-health-and-welfare/
animal-welfare/

https://www.aspca.org/protecting-farm-animals/
problem-factory-farming

https://www.ncbi.nlm.nih.gov/pmc/articles/PMC9757169/

SLEEP

How Drunk Are You Without Sleep?

https://www.nmt.edu/cds/
How_Drunk_Are_You_Without_Sleep.pdf

Meal planning template

Sunday

Breakfast -

Lunch -

Dinner -

Monday

Breakfast -

Lunch -

Dinner -

Tuesday

Breakfast -

Lunch -

Dinner –

Wednesday

Breakfast -

Lunch -

Dinner –

Thursday

Breakfast -

Lunch -

Dinner -

Friday

Breakfast -

Lunch -

Dinner -

Saturday

Breakfast -

Lunch -

Dinner -

Grocery List Template

Produce Section

Meat Section

Refrigerated Section

Frozen Section

Aisles

Non-Food Products

Citations

For convenient access to these citations, visit https://www.barbaraalifdoran.com.

[1] Medscape Physician Compensation Report 2017; https://www.amnhealthcare.com/blog/physician/locums/average-time-doctors-spend-with-patients/

[2] Neprash, HT et al; Association of Primary Care Visit Length With Potentially Inappropriate Prescribing, *JAMA Health Forum.* 2023;4(3):e230052; https://jamanetwork.com/journals/jama-health-forum/fullarticle/2802144

[3] Adult Immunization Schedule by Age; addendum jupdated June 27, 2024; CDC; https://www.cdc.gov/vaccines/schedules/hcp/imz/adult.html

[4] McDowell R et al, Oral antibiotic use and early-onset colorectal cancer: findings from a case-control study using a national clinical database; British Journal of Cancer; 17 December 2021; https://www.nature.com/articles/s41416-021-01665-7

[5] Emergency Physicians.org; Know When to GO; https://www.emergencyphysicians.org/article/know-when-to-go/know-when-to-go-overview

[6] Basu g, et al; Clinicians' Obligations to Use Qualified Medical Interpreters When Caring for Patients with Limited English Proficiency; AMA Journal of Ethics®, March 2017; https://journalofethics.ama-assn.org/article/clinicians-obligations-

190

use-qualified-medical-interpreters-when-caring-patients-limited-english/2017-03

[7] Assistant Secretary for Planning and Evaluation, Officer of Health Policy, https://aspe.hhs.gov/sites/default/files/documents/ e497c623e5a0216b31291cd37063df1d/NHIS-Q3-2023-Data-Point-FINAL.pdf; Data Point, HP-2024-02

[8] The Commonwealth Fund; The State of U.S. Health Insurance in 2002; https://www.commonwealthfund.org/publications/issue-briefs/2022/sep/state-us-health-insurance-2022-biennial-survey

[9] Young Adults and the Affordable Care Act: Protecting Young Adults and Eliminating Burdens on Businesses and Families FAQs; U.S. Department of Labor, Employee Benefits Security Administration; https://www.dol.gov/agencies/ebsa/about-ebsa/ our-activities/resource-center/faqs/young-adult-and-aca

[10] Harker L and Sharer B; Medicaid Expansion: Frequently Asked Questions; Center on Budget and Policy Priorities; June 14, 2024; https://www.cbpp.org/research/health/medicaid-expansion-frequently-asked-questions-0

[11] New Report: 40% of Older Americans Rely Solely on Social Security for Retirement Income; National Institute on Retirement Security; January 13, 2020; https://www.nirsonline.org/2020/01/ new-report-40-of-older-americans-rely-solely-on-social-security-for-retirement-income/

[12] https://www.medicare.gov/drug-coverage-part-d/how-to-get-prescription-drug-coverage

[13] The Office of the National Coordinator for Health Information Technology; The ONC Cures Act Final Rule;

https://www.healthit.gov/sites/default/files/page2/2020-03/
TheONCCuresActFinalRule.pdf

[14] Office of the Comptroller of the Currency; Financial Literacy Resource Directory; https://www.occ.gov/topics/consumers-and-communities/community-affairs/resource-directories/financial-literacy/index-financial-literacy-resource-directory.html

[15] Reynolds S, FDA Approves HPV Tests That Allow for Self-Collection in a Health Care Setting; National Cancer Institute; July 24, 2024; https://www.cancer.gov/news-events/cancer-currents-blog/2024/fda-hpv-test-self-collection-health-care-setting

[16] American Cancer Society Statement: FDA Approval of HPV Self-Collection for Cervical Cancer Screening; American Cancer Society, May 15, 2024; https://pressroom.cancer.org/releases?item=1325

[17] Yedjou CG et al; Health and Racial Disparity in Breast Cancer, Adv Exp Med Biol. 2019; 1152: 31–49; https://www.ncbi.nlm.nih.gov/pmc/articles/PMC6941147/#[1]

[18] National Cancer Institute Staff; Why is Colorectal Cancer Rising Rapidly Among Young Adults?; November 5, 2020; https://www.cancer.gov/news-events/cancer-currents-blog/2020/colorectal-cancer-rising-younger-adults

[19] Collins S; 2024—First Year the US Expects More than 2M New Cases of Cancer; American Cancer Society; January 17, 2024; https://www.cancer.org/research/acs-research-news/facts-and-figures-2024.html#[2]

---

1. https://www.ncbi.nlm.nih.gov/pmc/articles/PMC6941147/

2. https://www.cancer.org/research/acs-research-news/facts-and-figures-2024.html

[20] Sung H et al; Differences in cancer rates among adults born between 1920 and 1990 in the USA: an analysis of population-based cancer registry data; The Lancet Public Health; Vol 9, Issue 8, E583-E593, August 2024

[21] Fry R et al, In a Growing Share of U.S. Marriages, Husbands and Wives Earn About the Same, Pew Research Center, April 13, 2023; https://www.pewresearch.org/social-trends/2023/04/13/in-a-growing-share-of-u-s-marriages-husbands-and-wives-earn-about-the-same/

[22] Wilding JPH et al, Once-Weekly Semaglutide in Adults with Overweight or Obesity, The New England Journal of Medicine, February 10, 2021; https://www.nejm.org/doi/full/10.1056/NEJMoa2032183

[23] Our World Data; Per capita meat consumption by type, 1961 to 2021; https://ourworldindata.org/grapher/per-capita-meat-consumption-by-type-kilograms-per-year?country=OWID_WRL~USA

[24] CDC, Heart Disease Facts; https://www.cdc.gov/heart-disease/data-research/facts-stats/?CDC_AAref_Val=https://www.cdc.gov/heartdisease/facts.htm

[25] Ahern K, Yes, you can fit exercise into a packed vacation—here's how, Johnson & Johnson, July 5, 2018

[26] Kianersi s et al, Association Between Accelerometer-Measured Irregular Sleep Duration and Type 2 Diabetes Risk: A Prospective Cohort Study in the UK Biobank; American Diabetes Association, July 17, 2024; https://doi.org/10.2337/dc24-0213

[27] Division of Sleep Medicine, Judgement and Safety, Harvard Medical School; https://sleep.hms.harvard.edu/education-training/

public-education/sleep-and-health-education-program/sleep-health-education-89#[3]

[28] National Heart. Lunch, and Blood Institute, How Sleep Affects your Health, https://www.nhlbi.nih.gov/health/sleep-deprivation/health-effects

Acknowledgements

With gratitude:

Paul, you have always supported me in pursuing my dreams, big and small. You believed in me more than I believed in myself to make those dreams a reality. Throughout our years of marriage, I have had many passion projects, and you never once told me that I couldn't make it happen. This is the first project where my dream came true!

Without my editor, Lisa Stockwell, this would have been another shelved passion project, but you took my words and created something that I never imagined possible. Because of you, this book will be an invaluable resource for all readers.

To all the amazing women who have been my patients, now or in the past, I want to express my heartfelt gratitude for giving me the privilege of being a part of your lives and for trusting me with your care, whether it was for a single visit or over many years. This book would not have been possible without you, and it's my gift to you, as it's hard to remember everything we talk about during a 20-minute appointment!

To my readers. I am grateful you bought this book and are committed to improving your health and well-being.